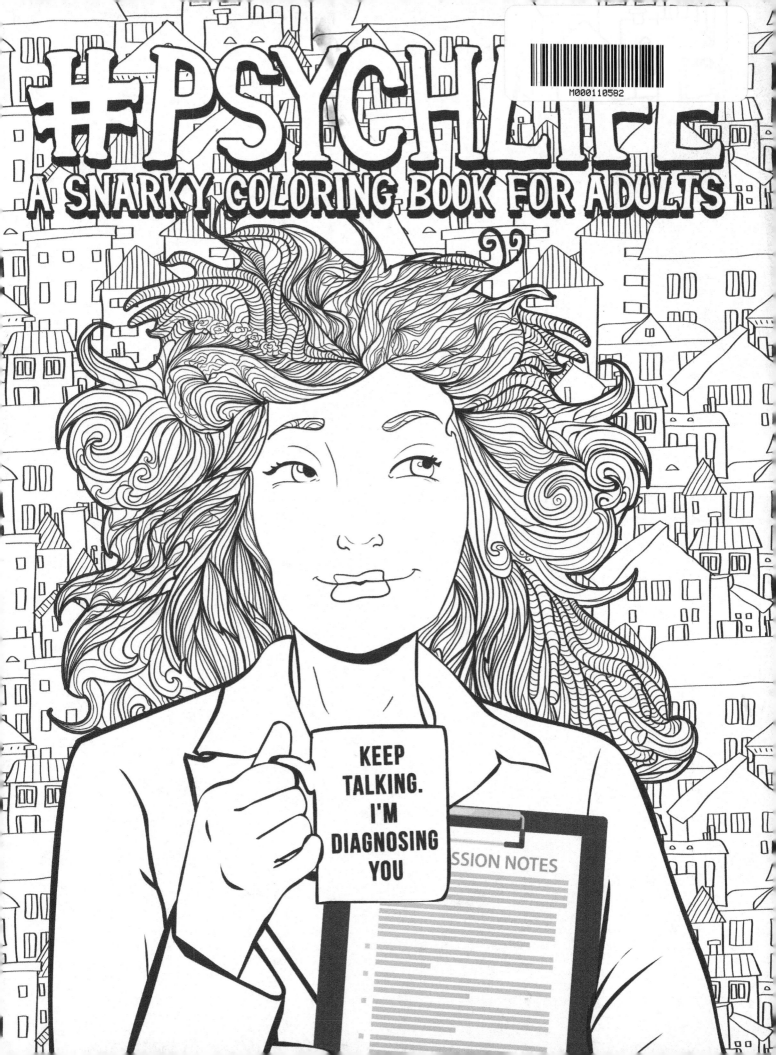

@papeteriebleu

Papeterie Bleu

Shop our other books at
www.pbleu.com

Wholesale distribution through Ingram Content Group
www.ingramcontent.com/publishers/distribution/wholesale

For questions and customer service, email us at
support@pbleu.com

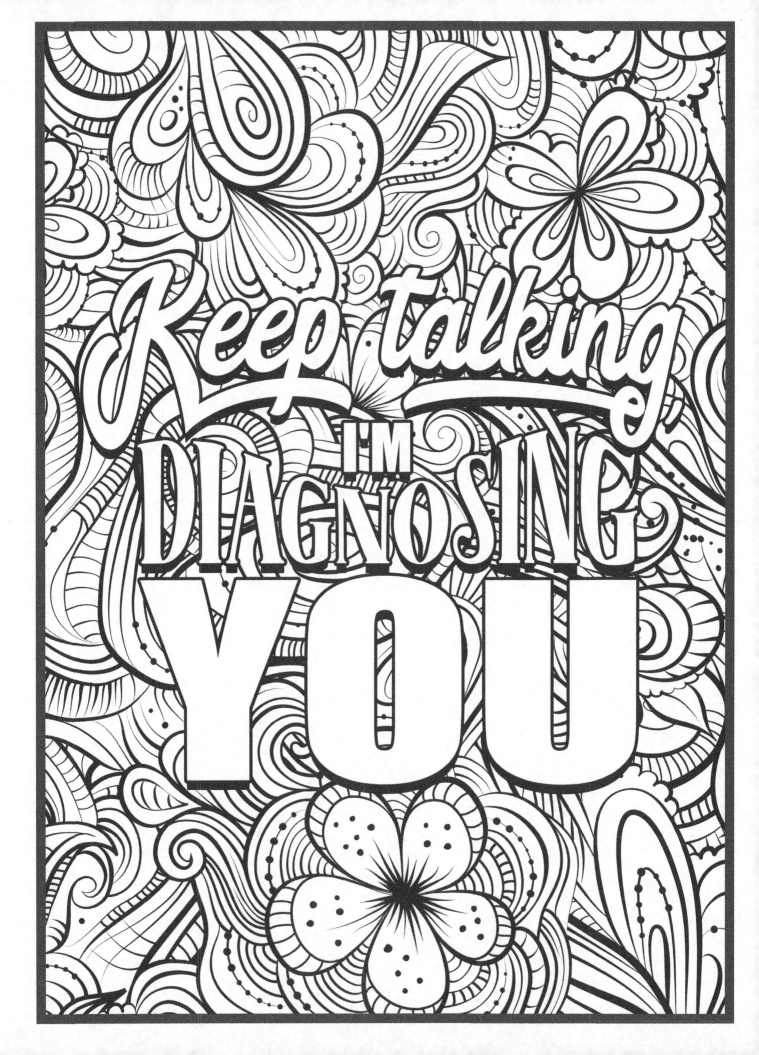

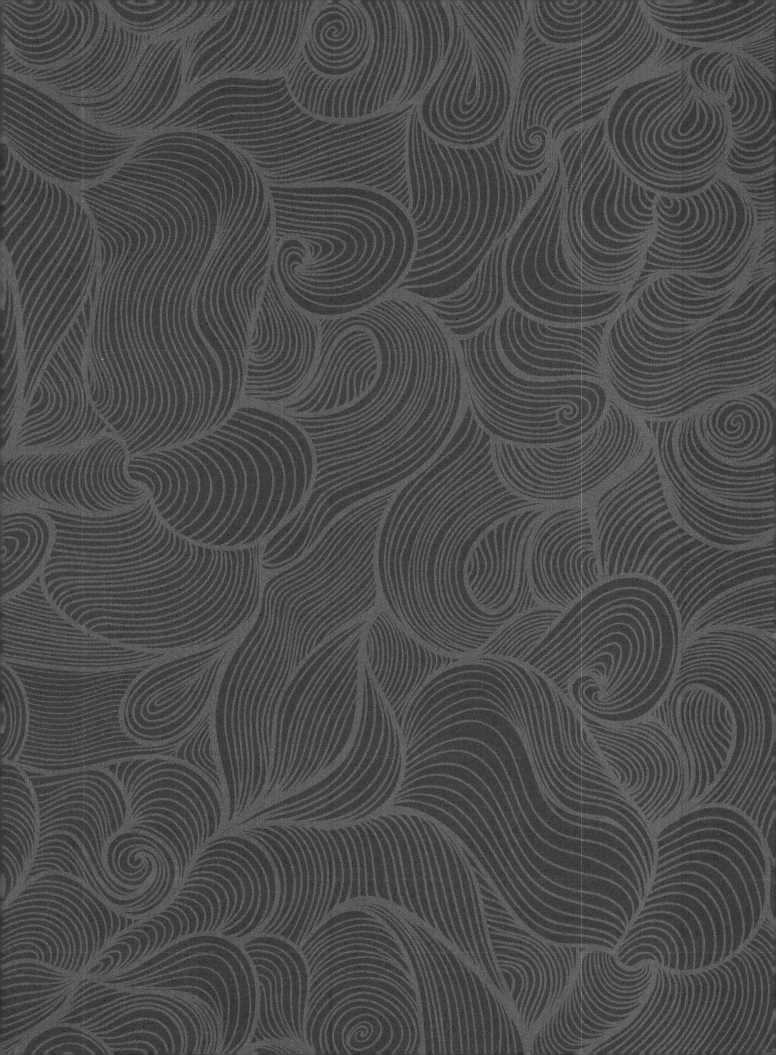

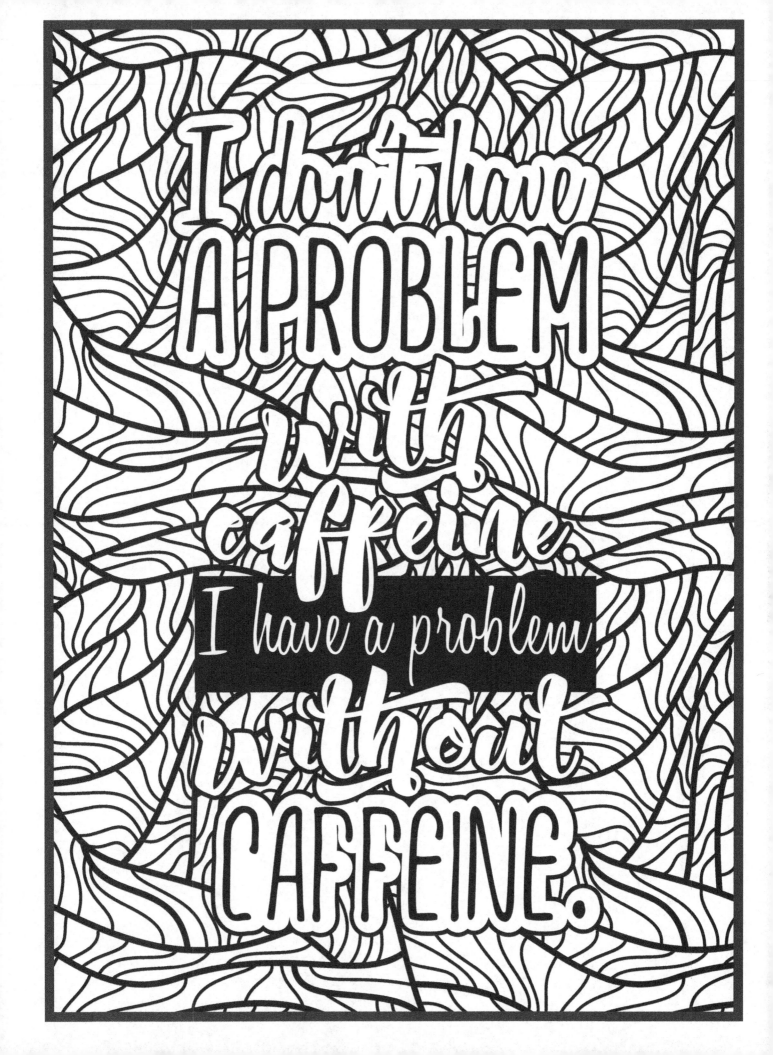

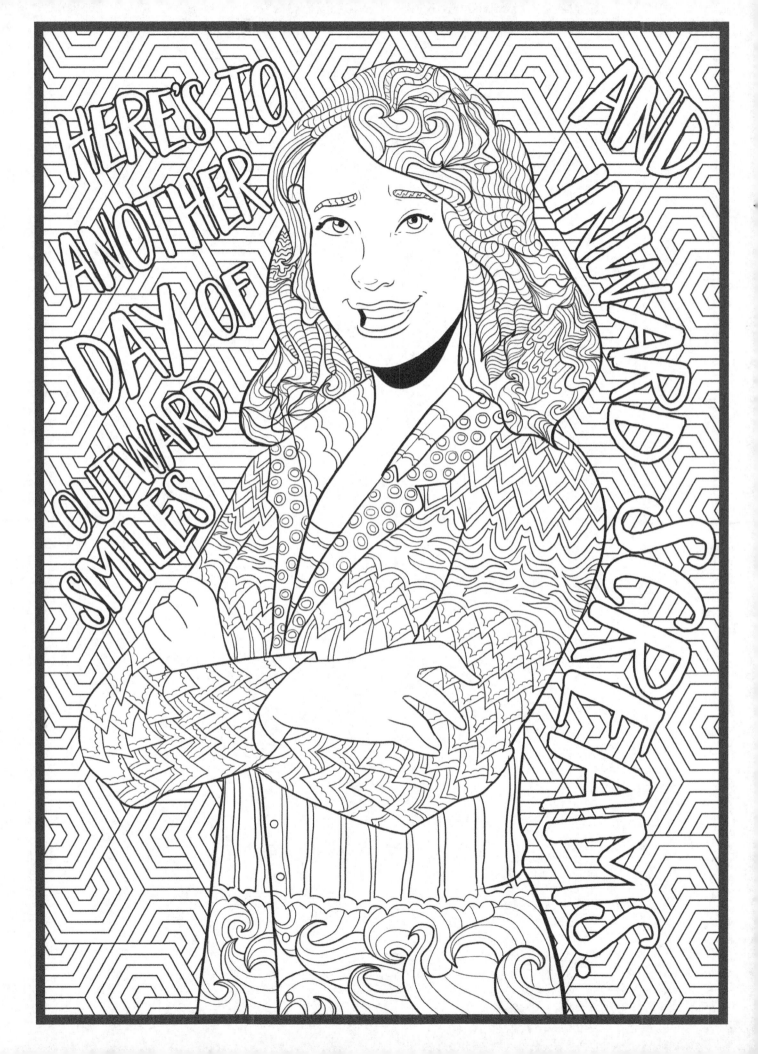

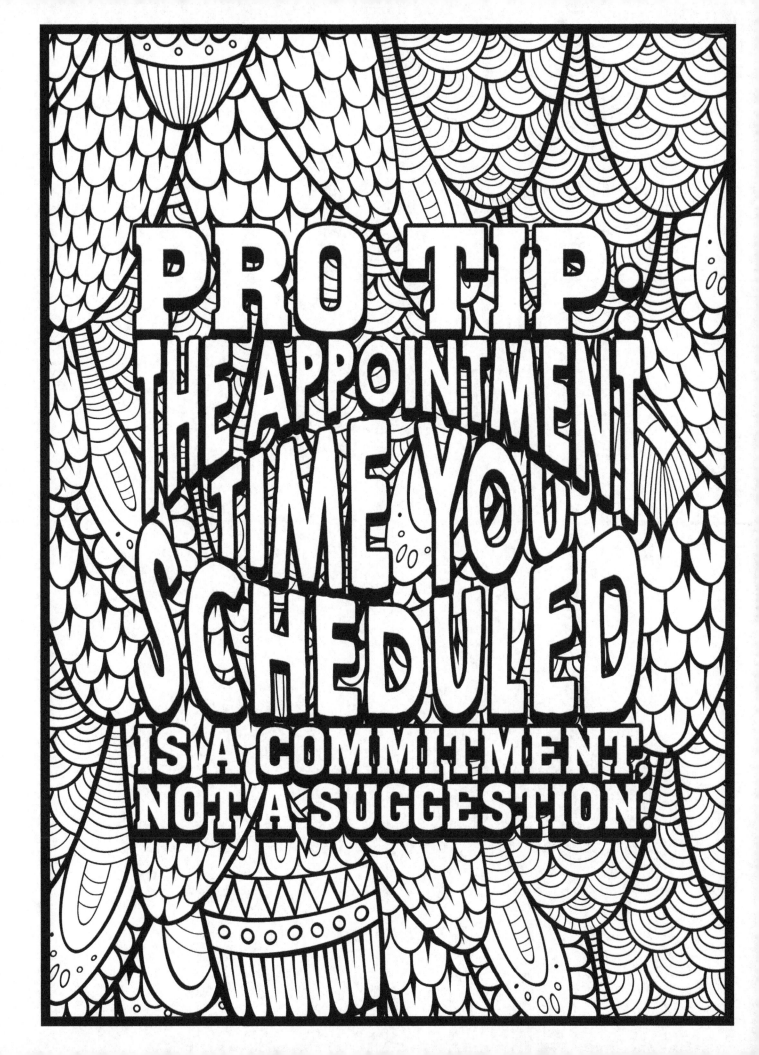

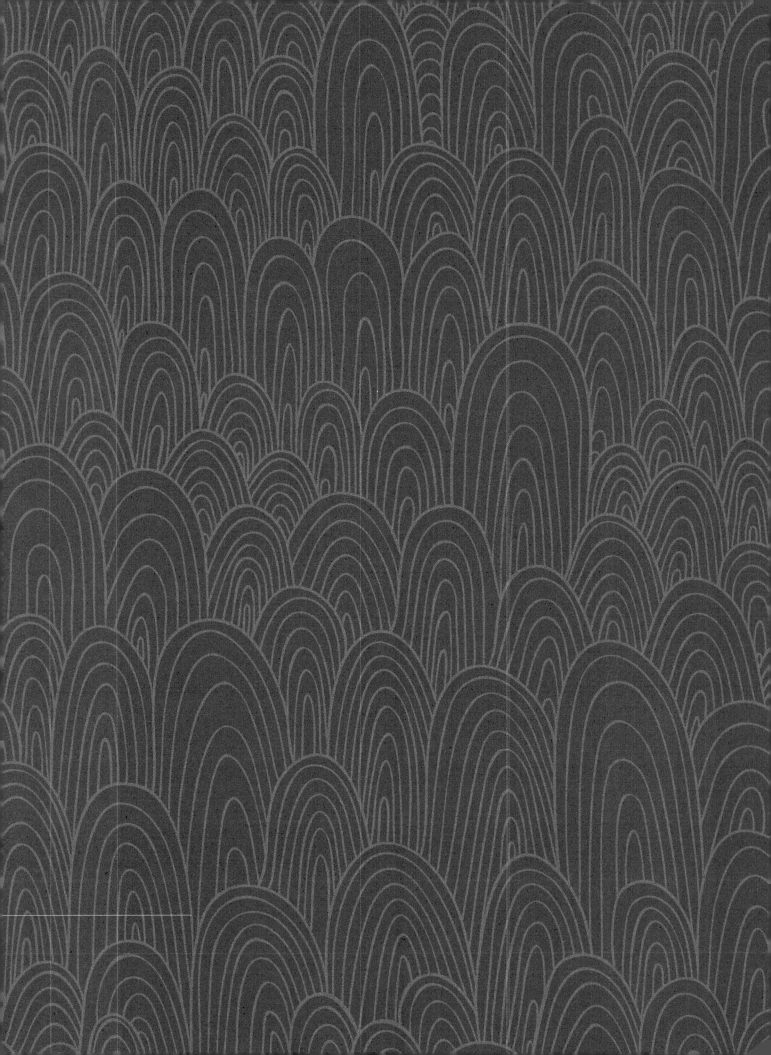

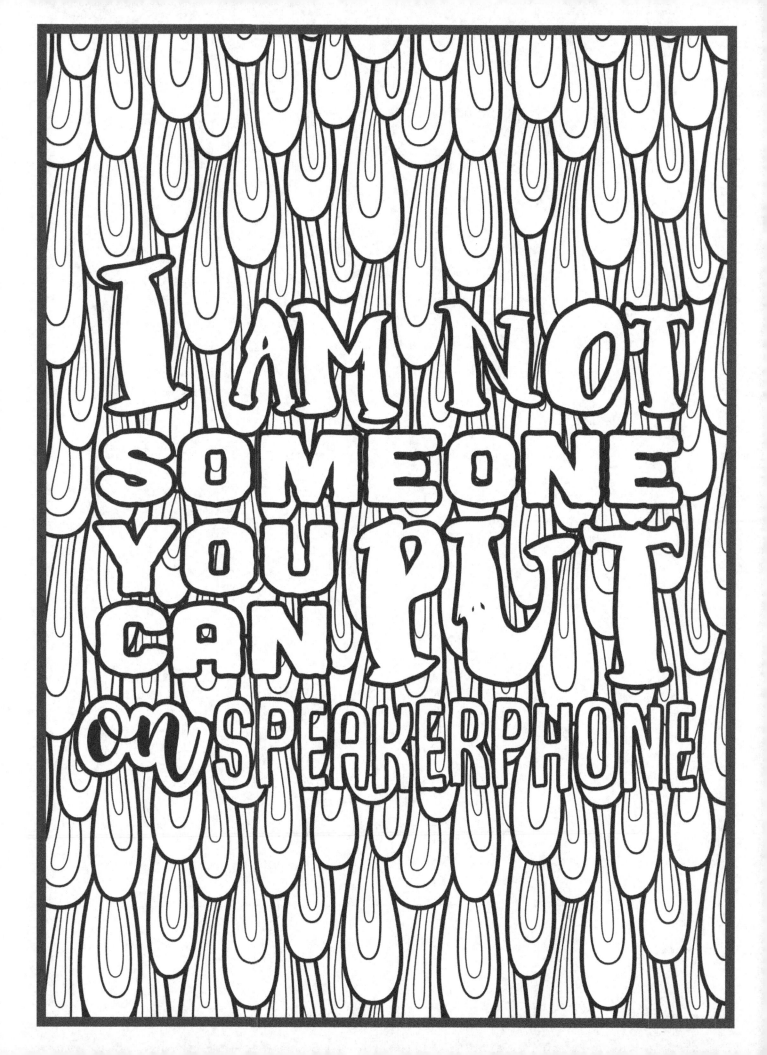

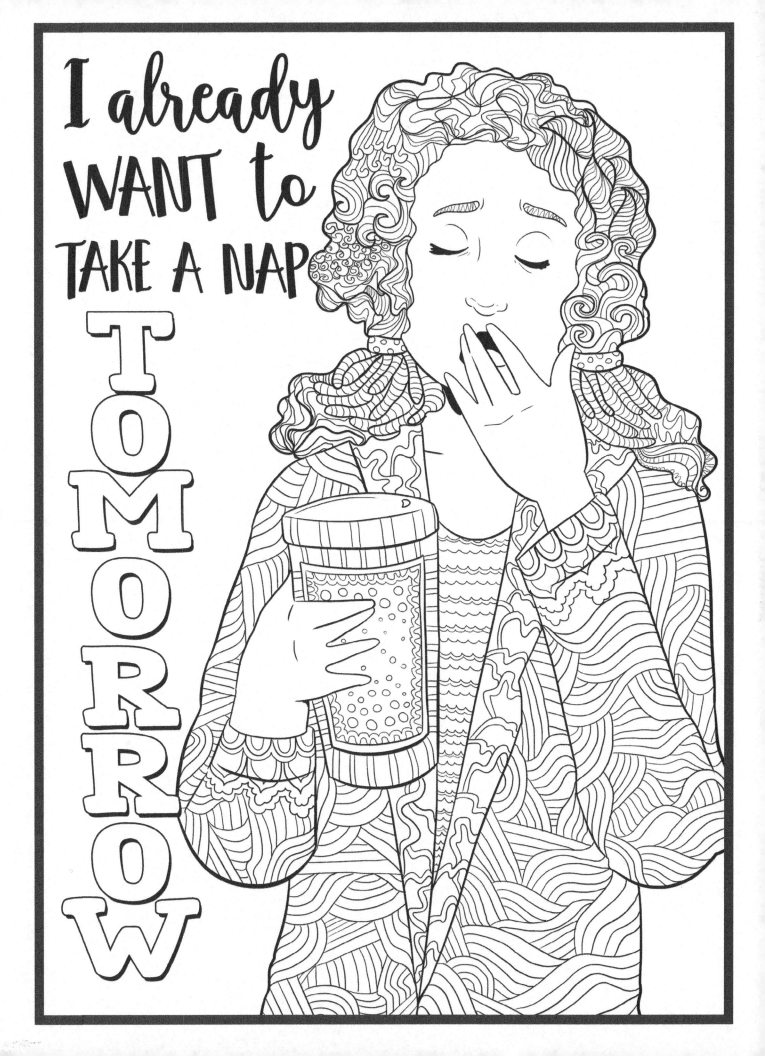

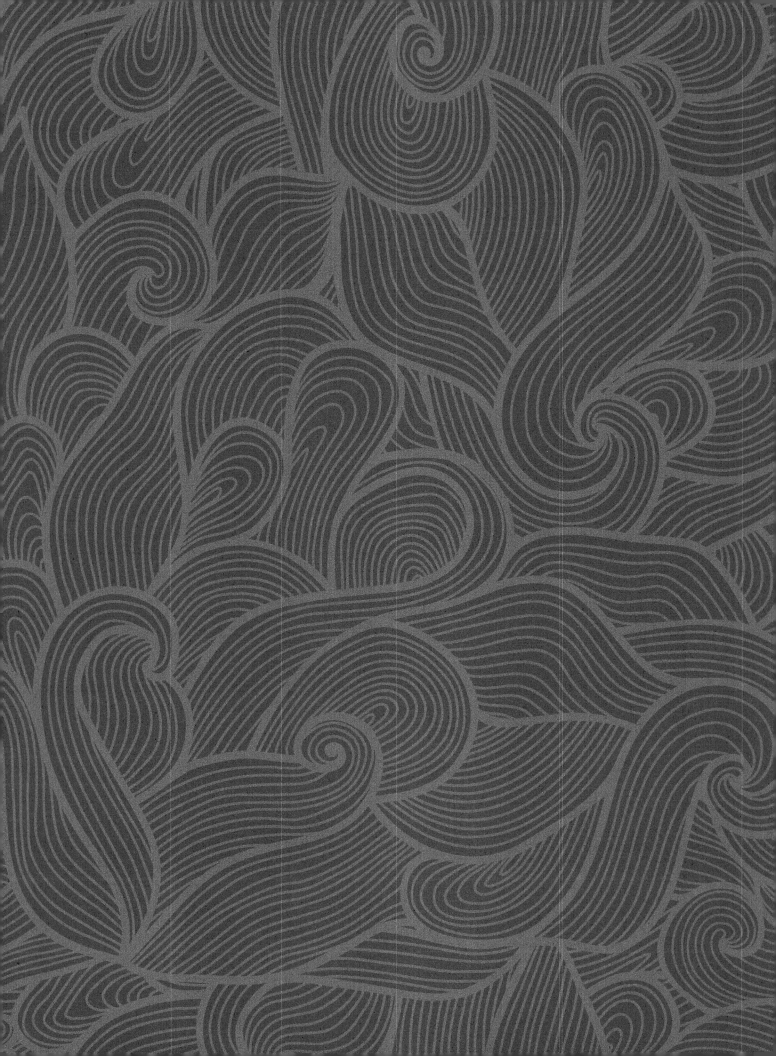

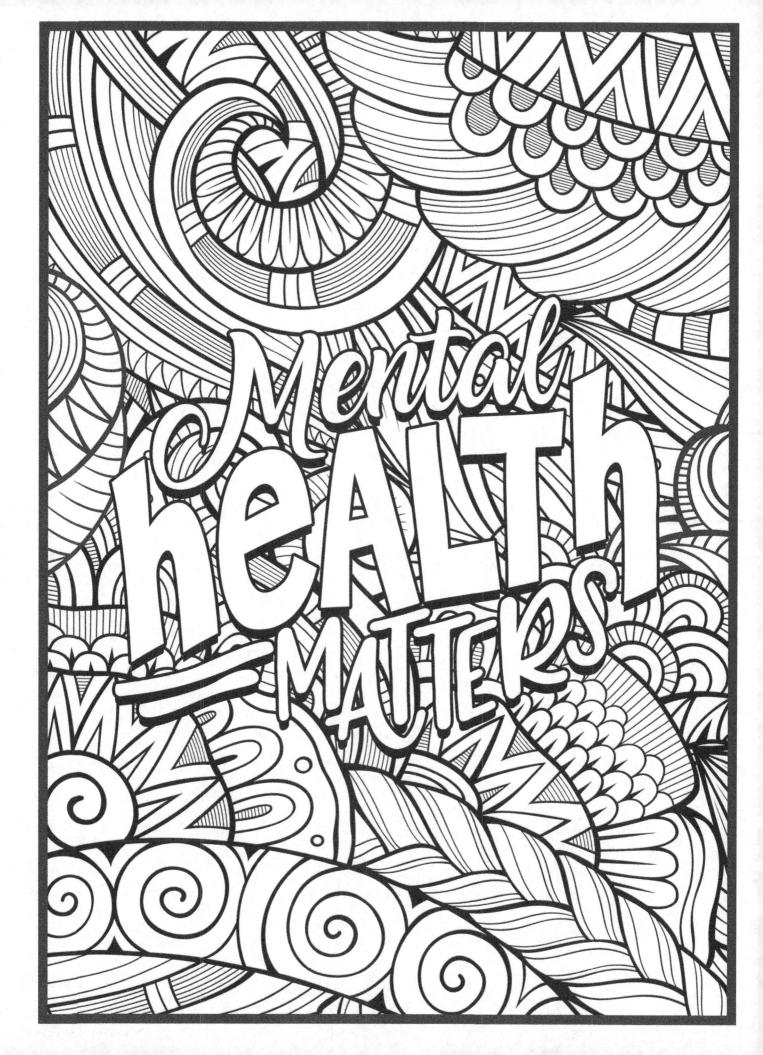

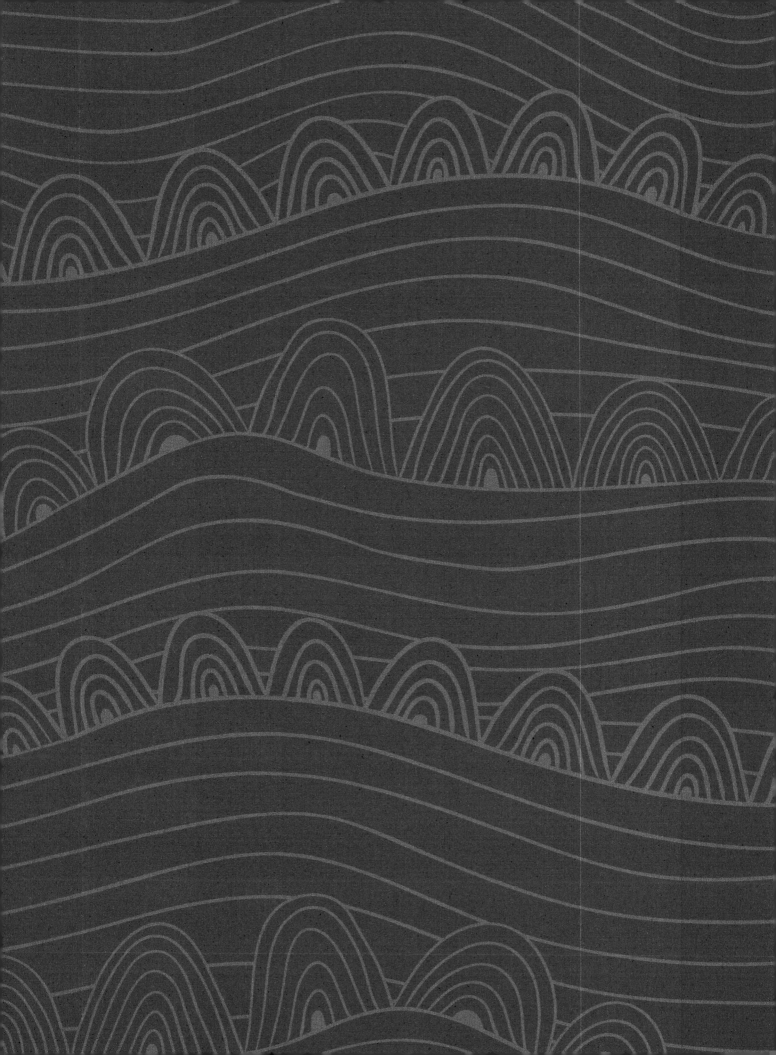

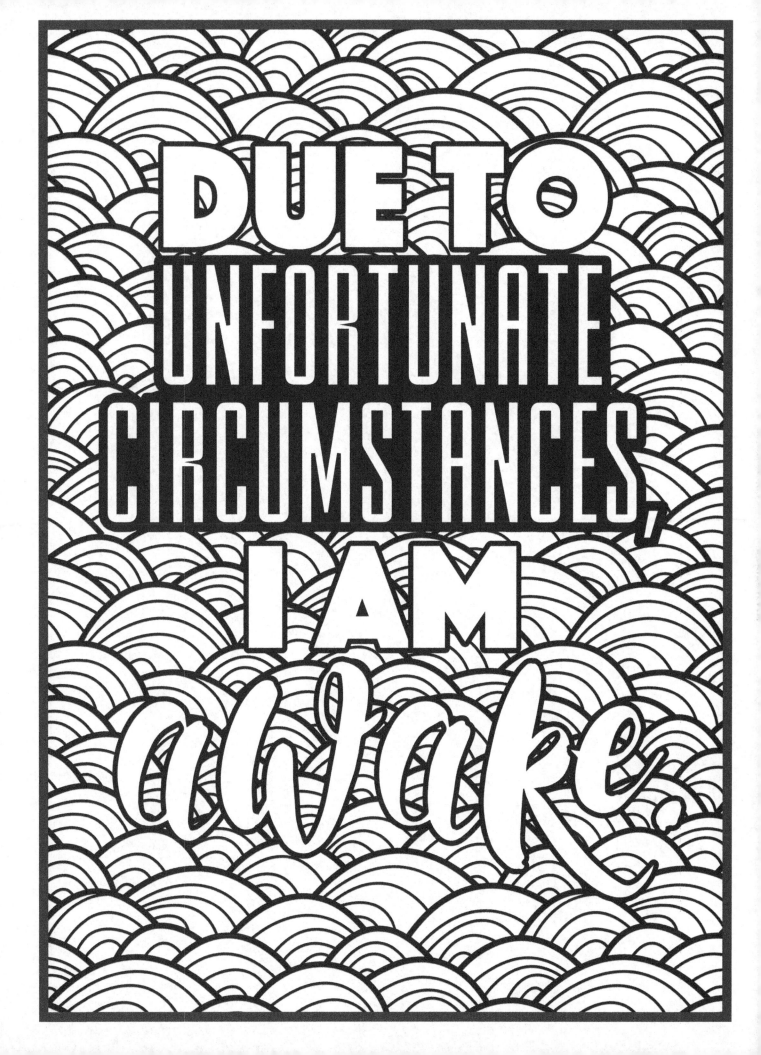

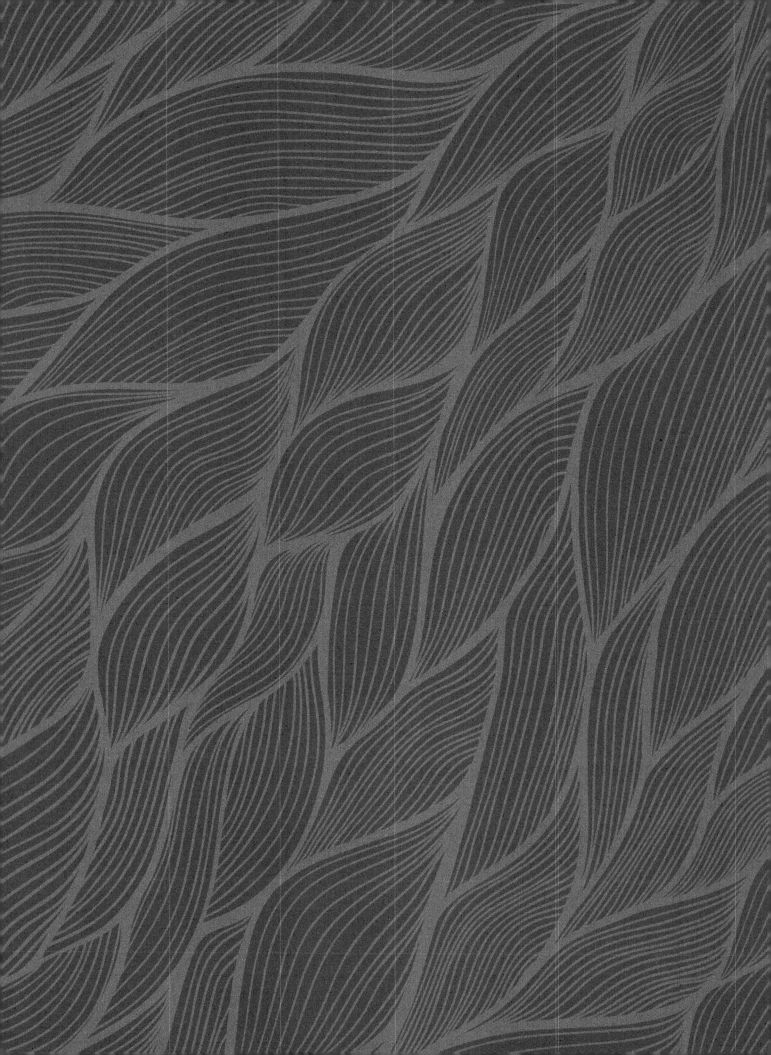

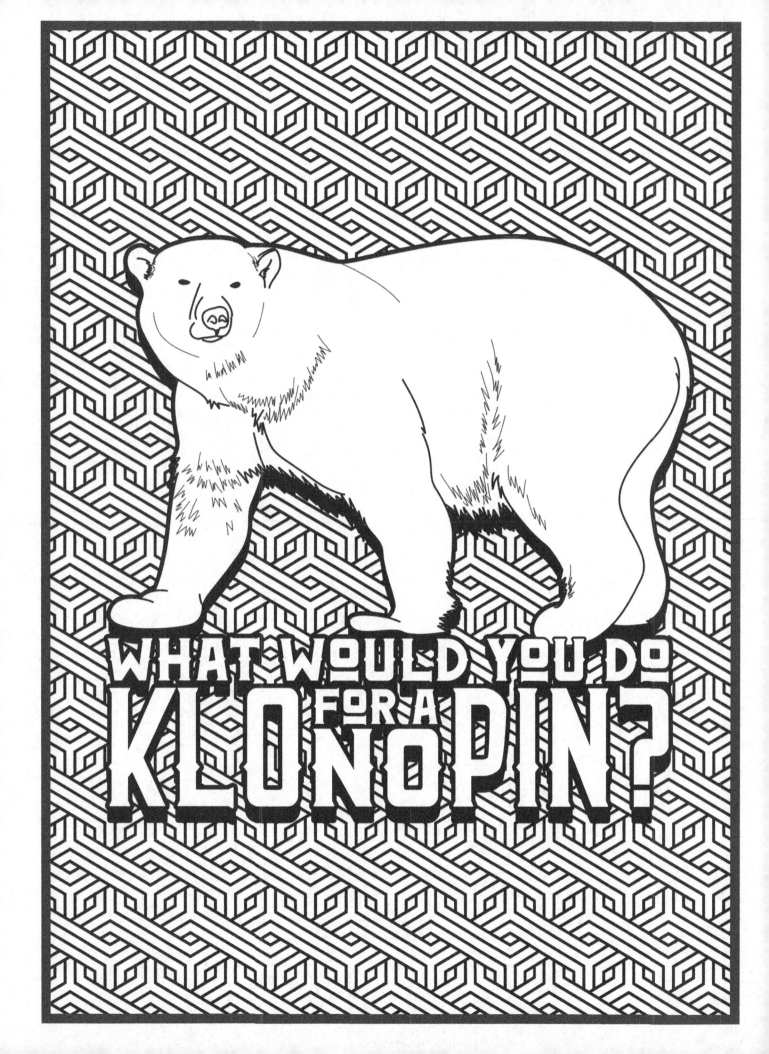

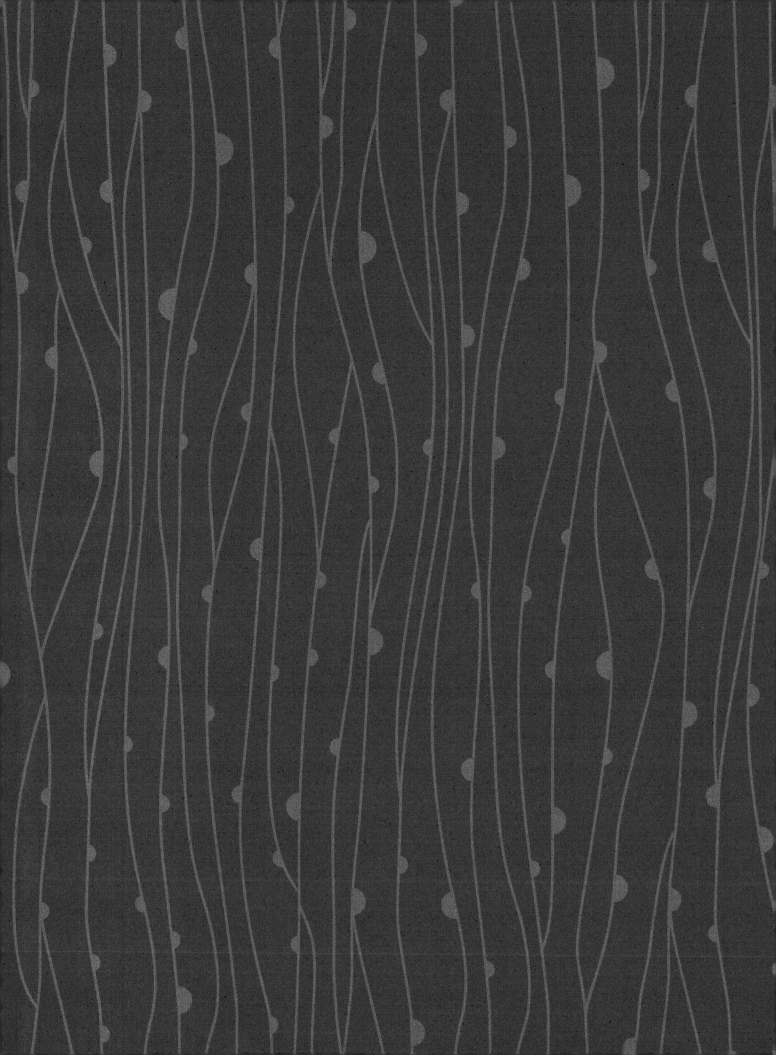

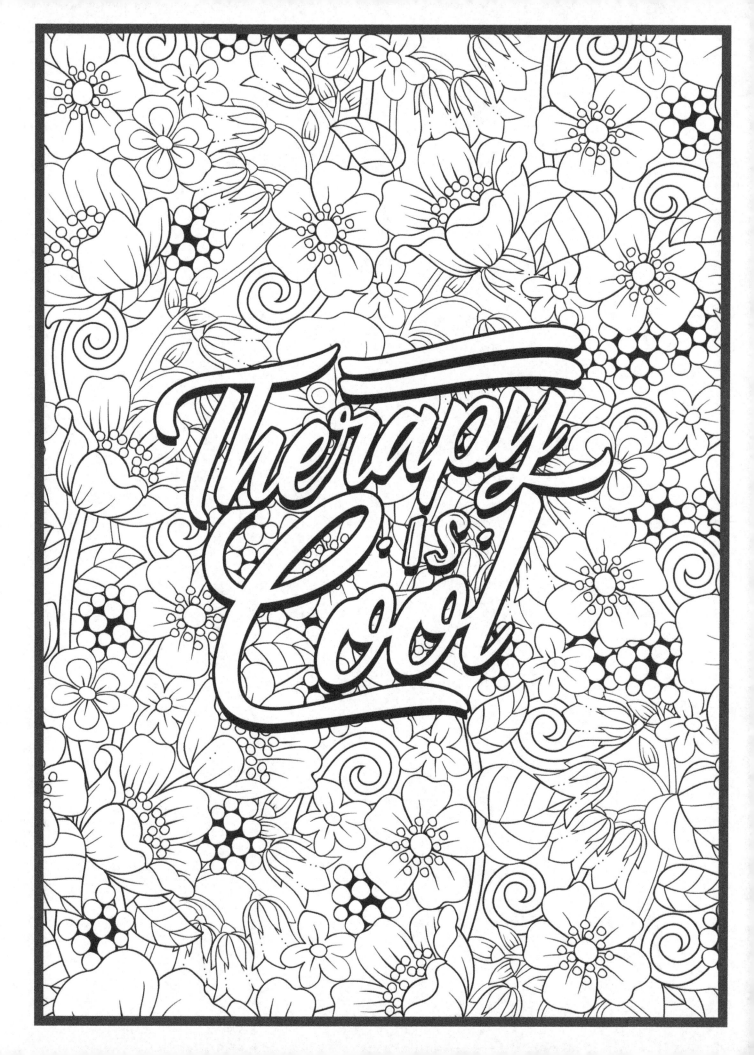

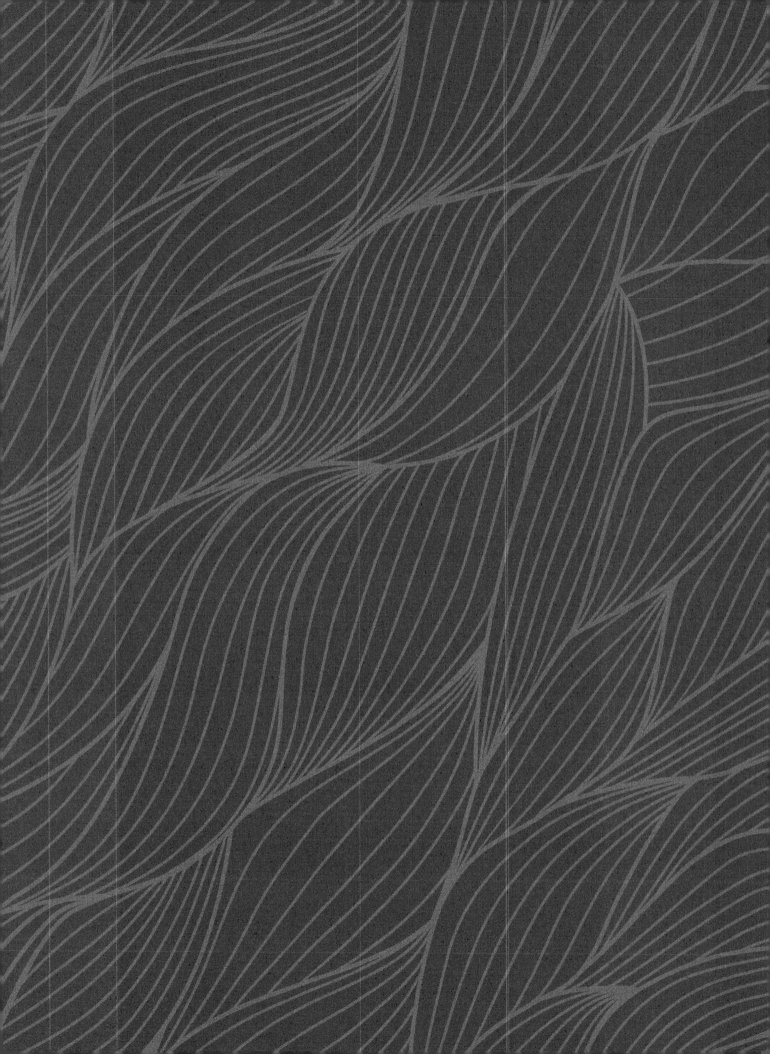

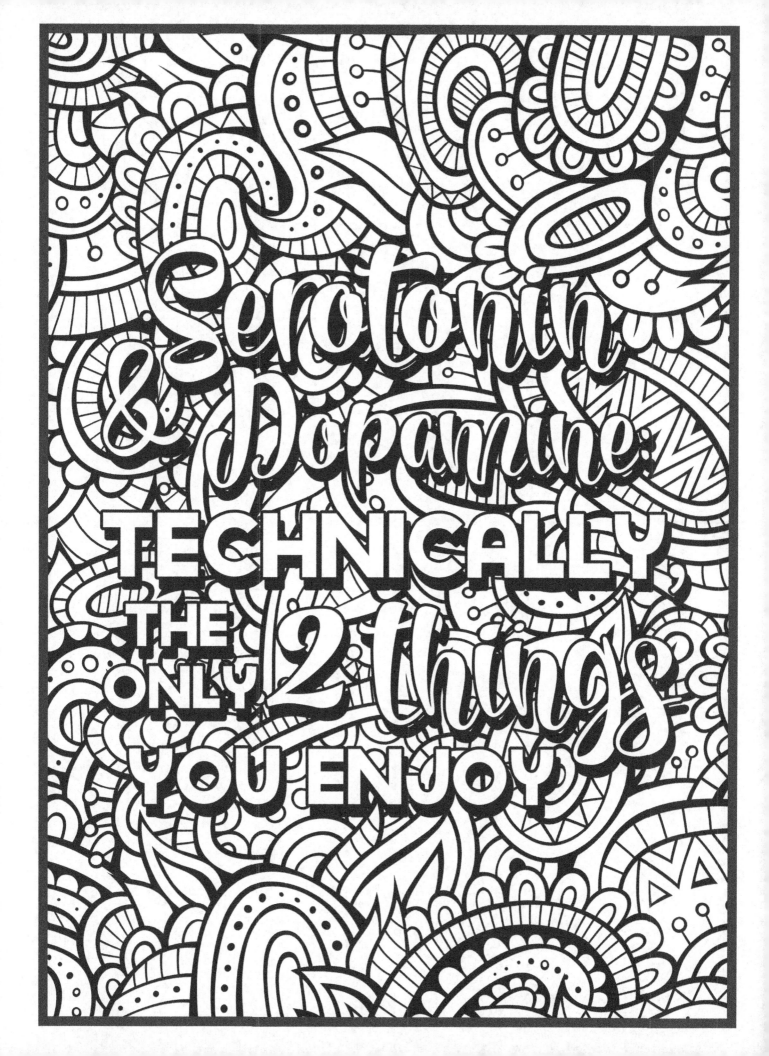

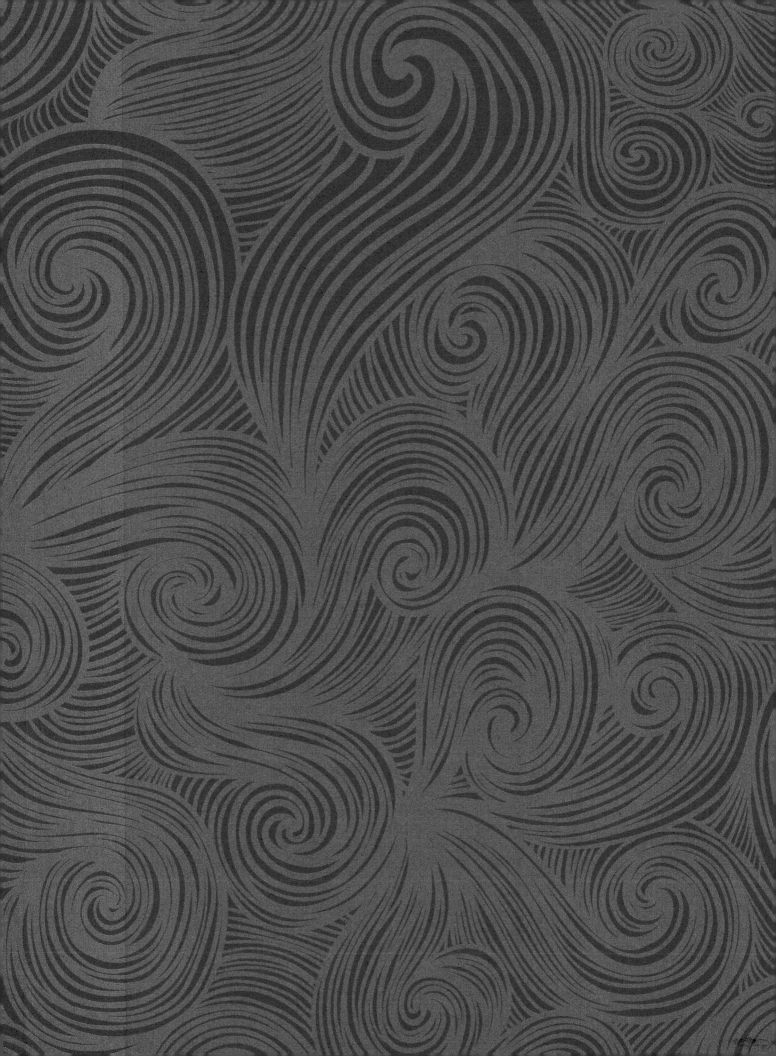

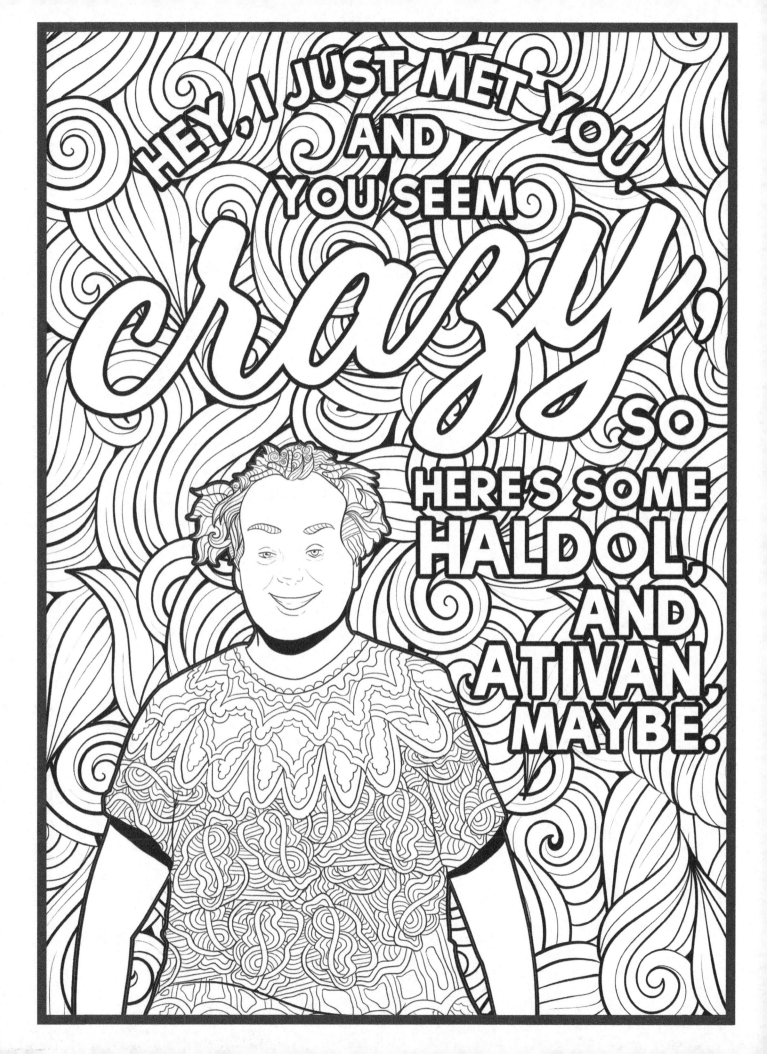

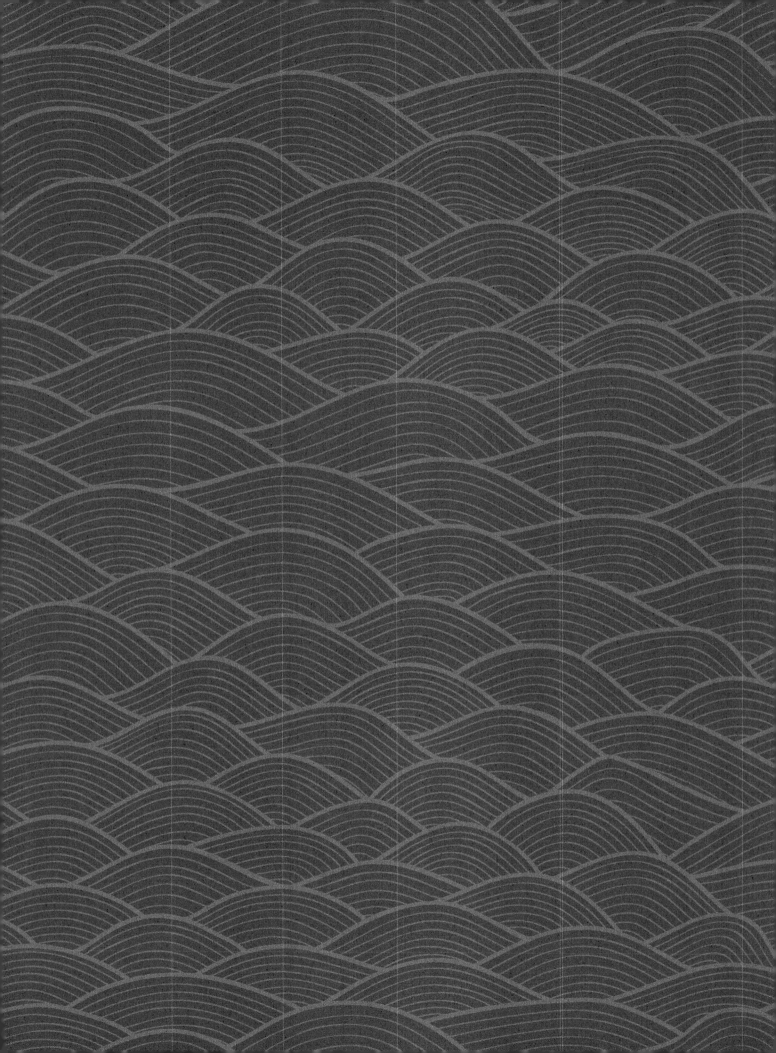

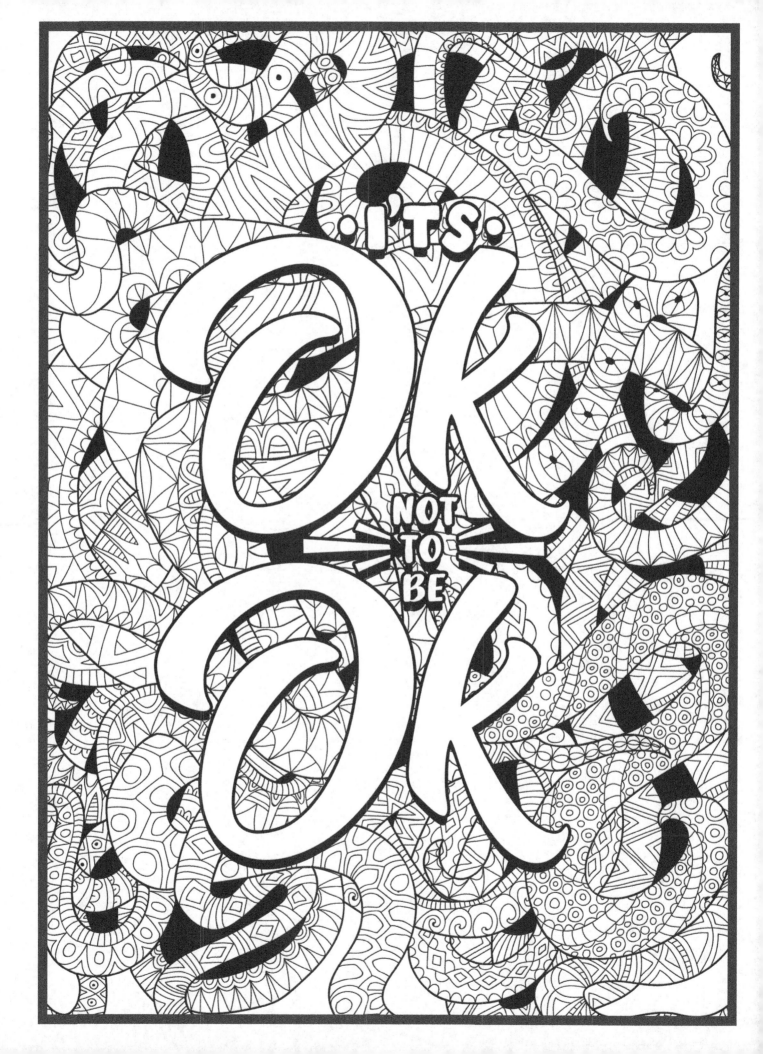

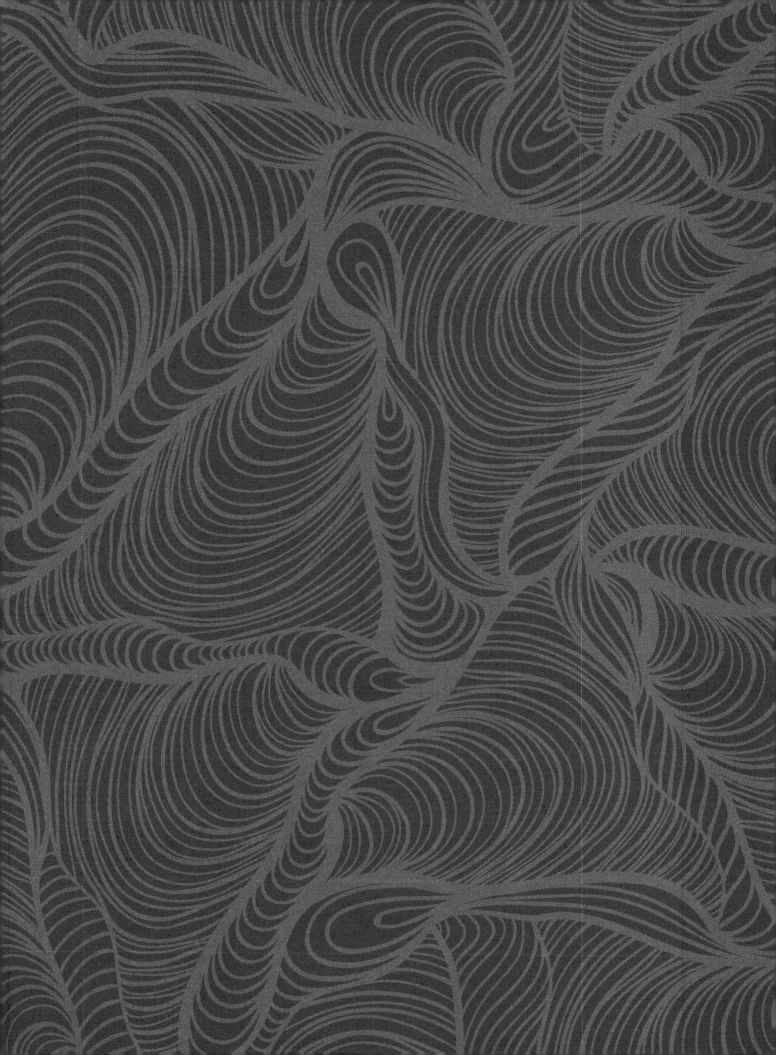

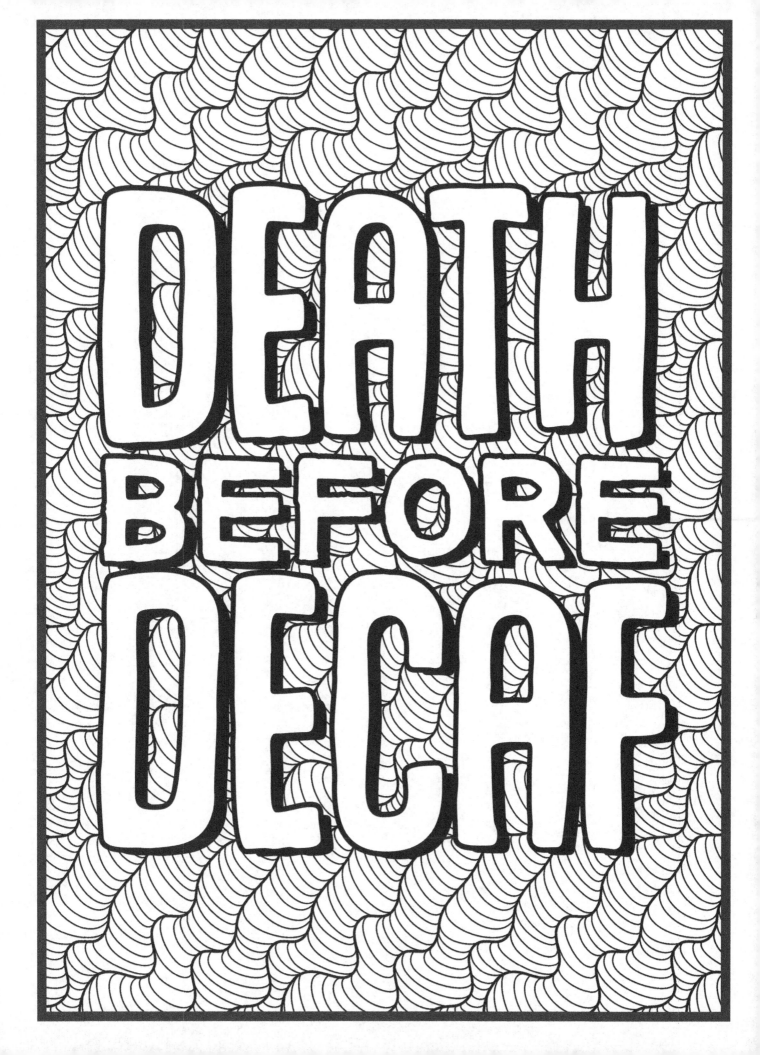

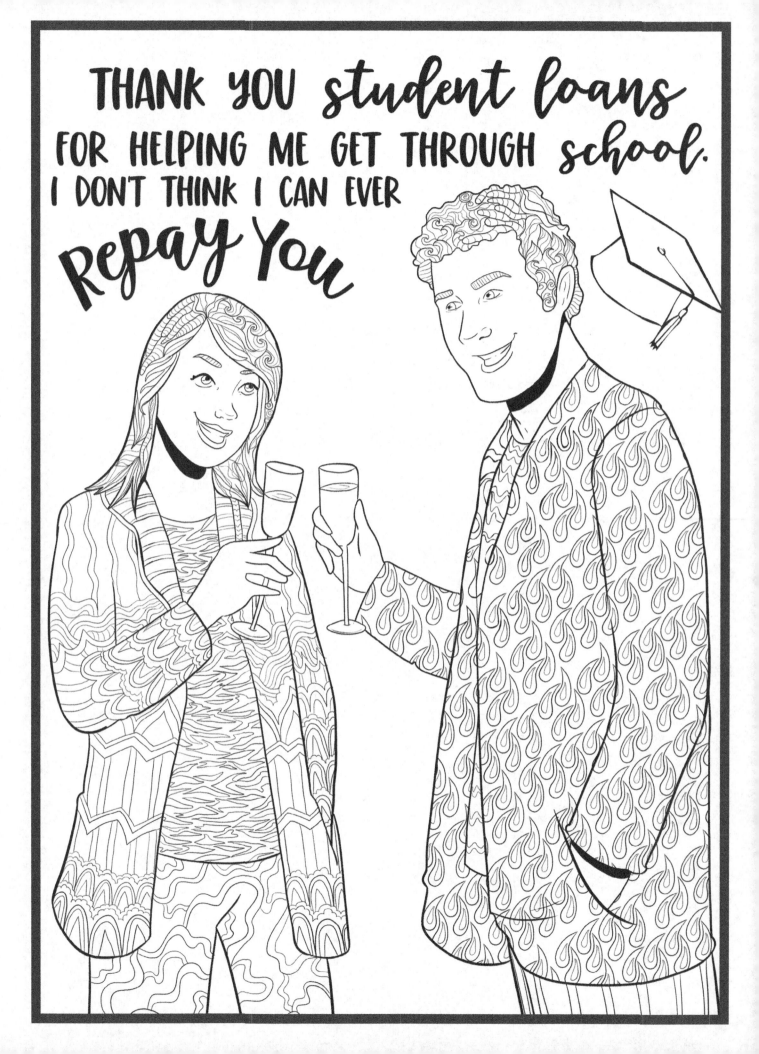

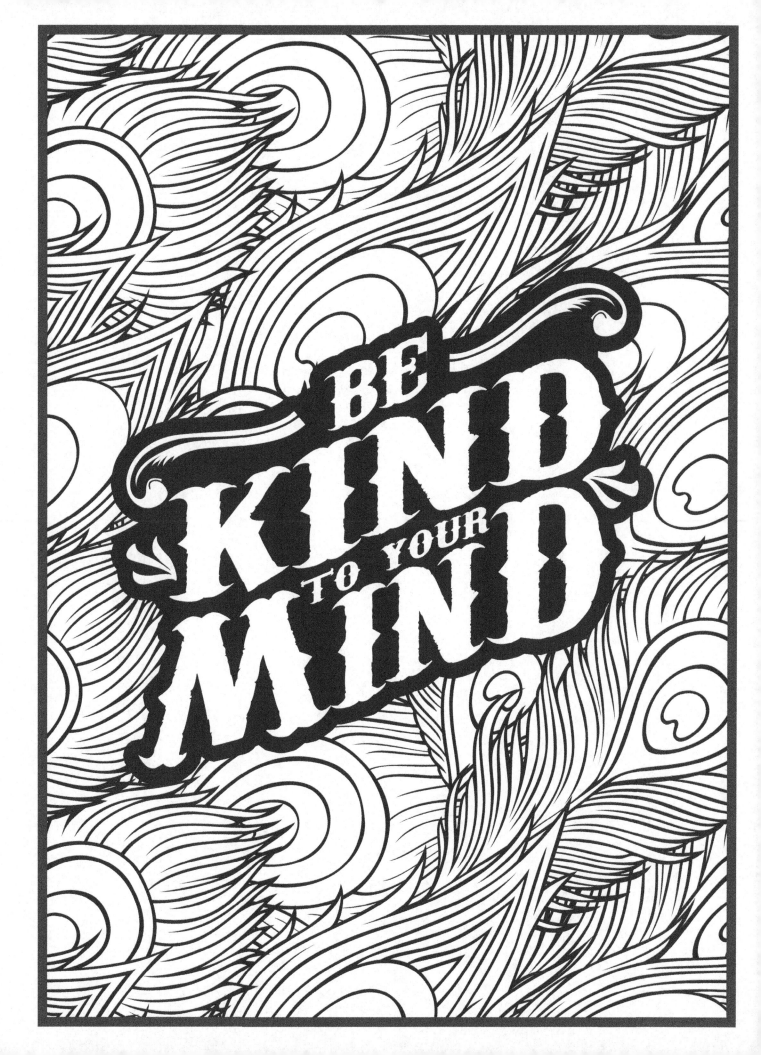

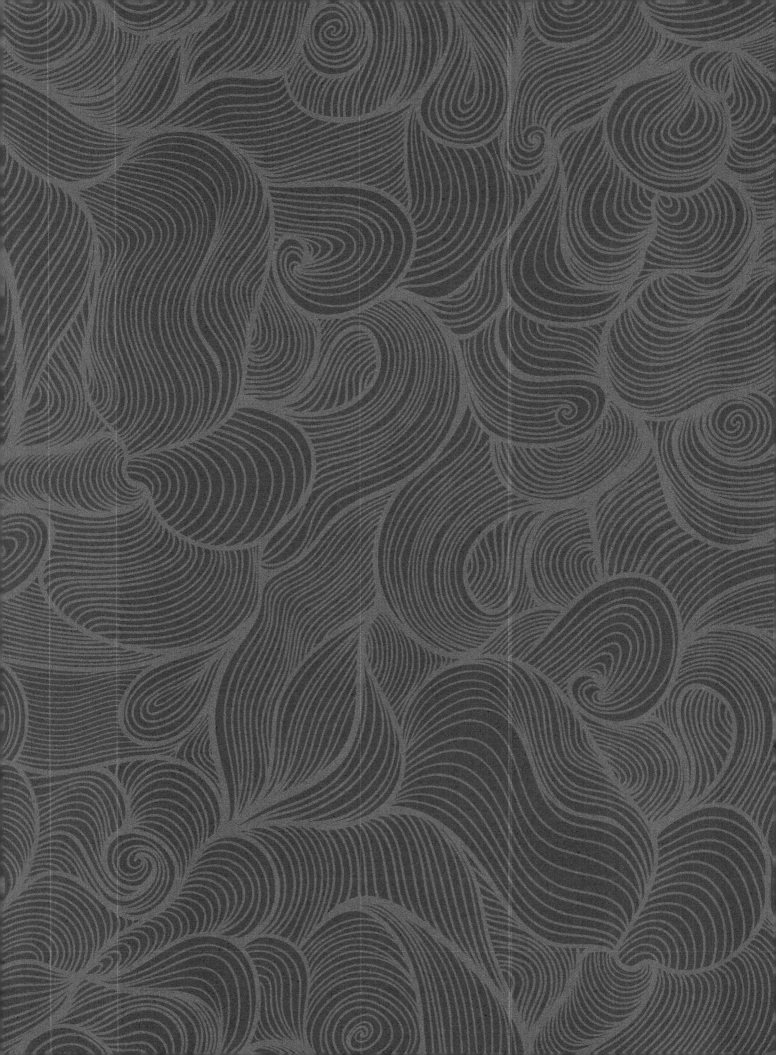

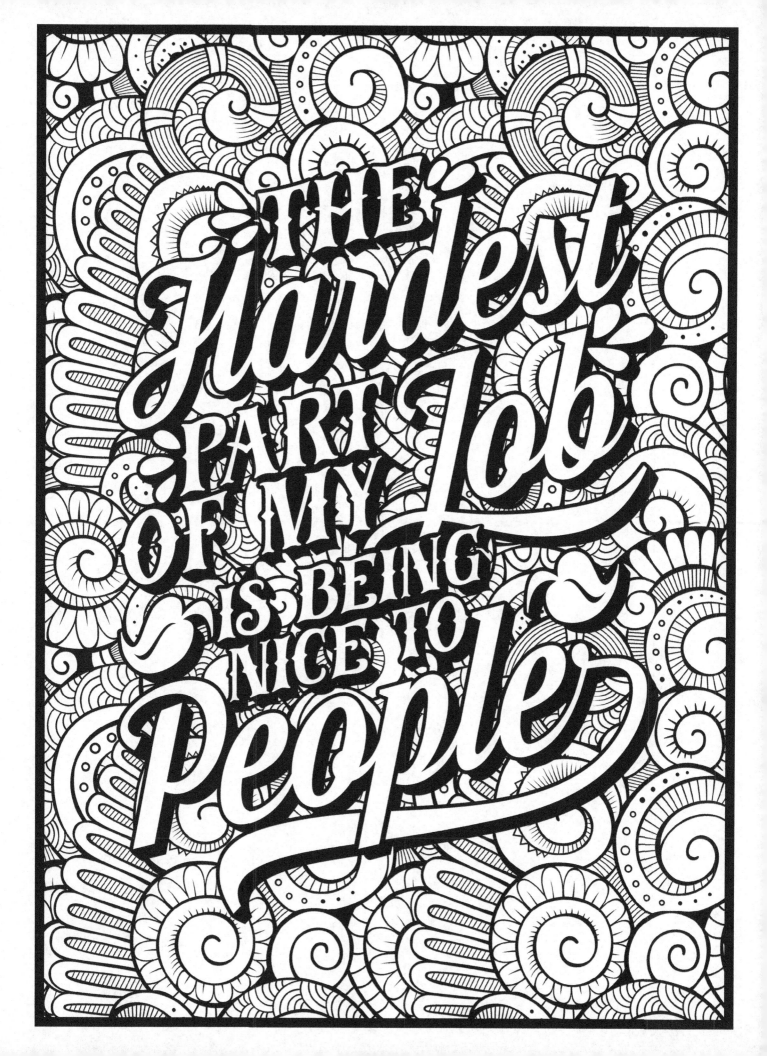

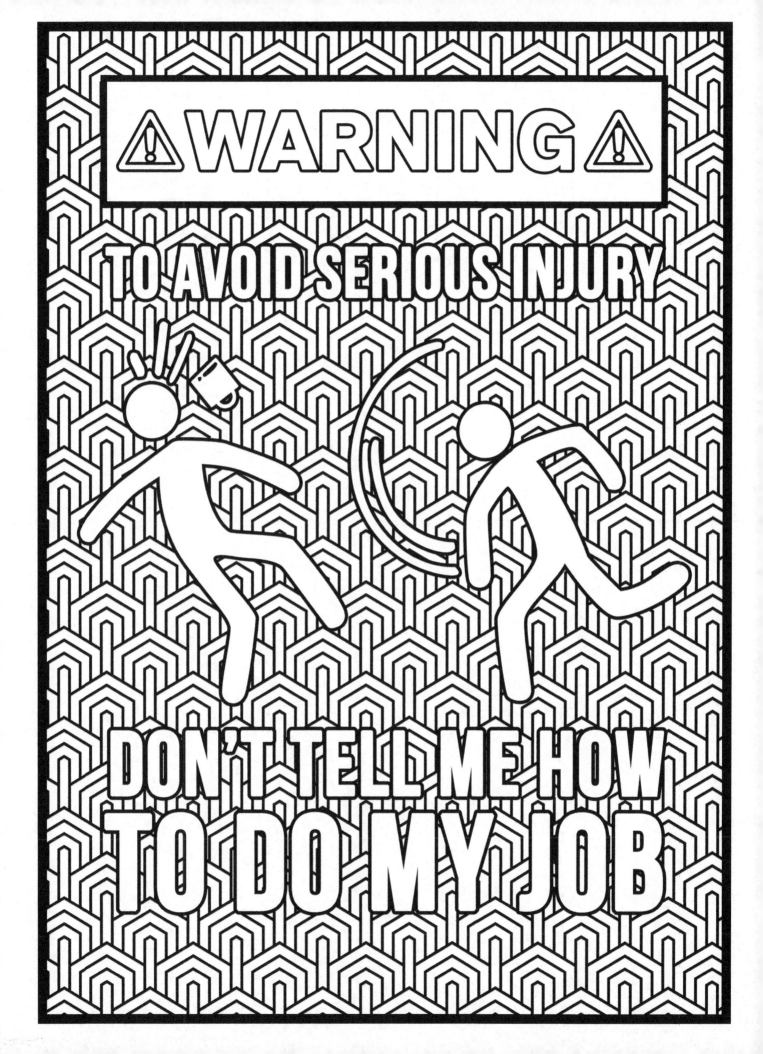

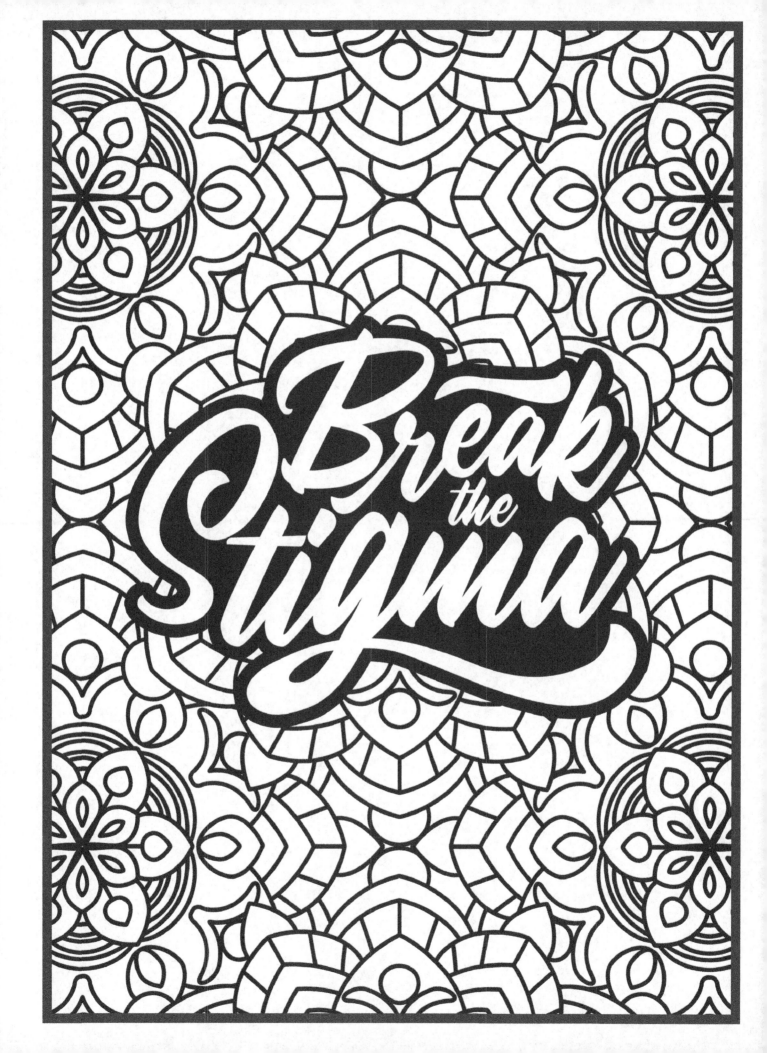

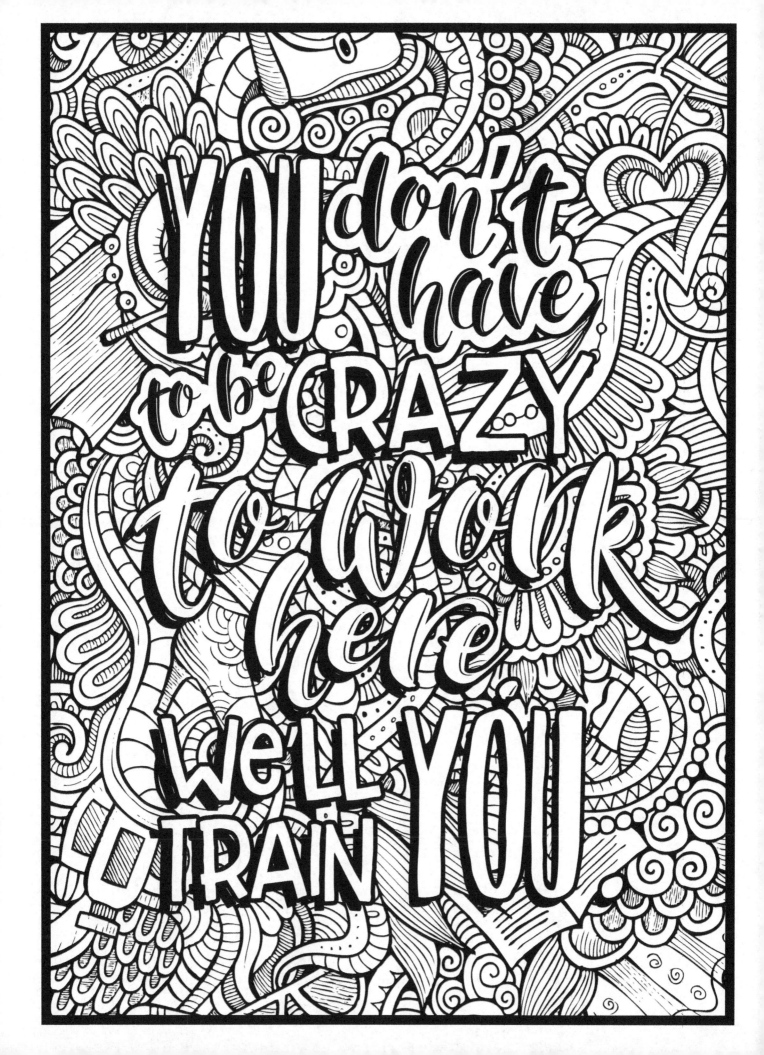

TECHNICALLY YOU'RE not DRINKING alone

if YOUR DOG is at home

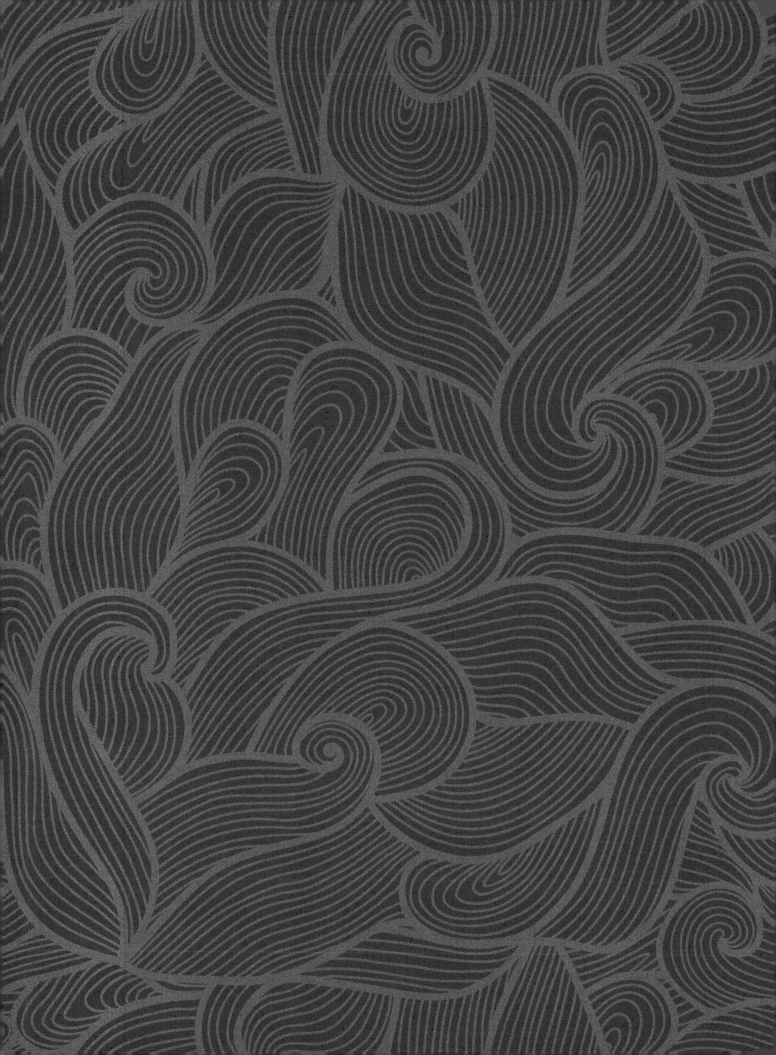

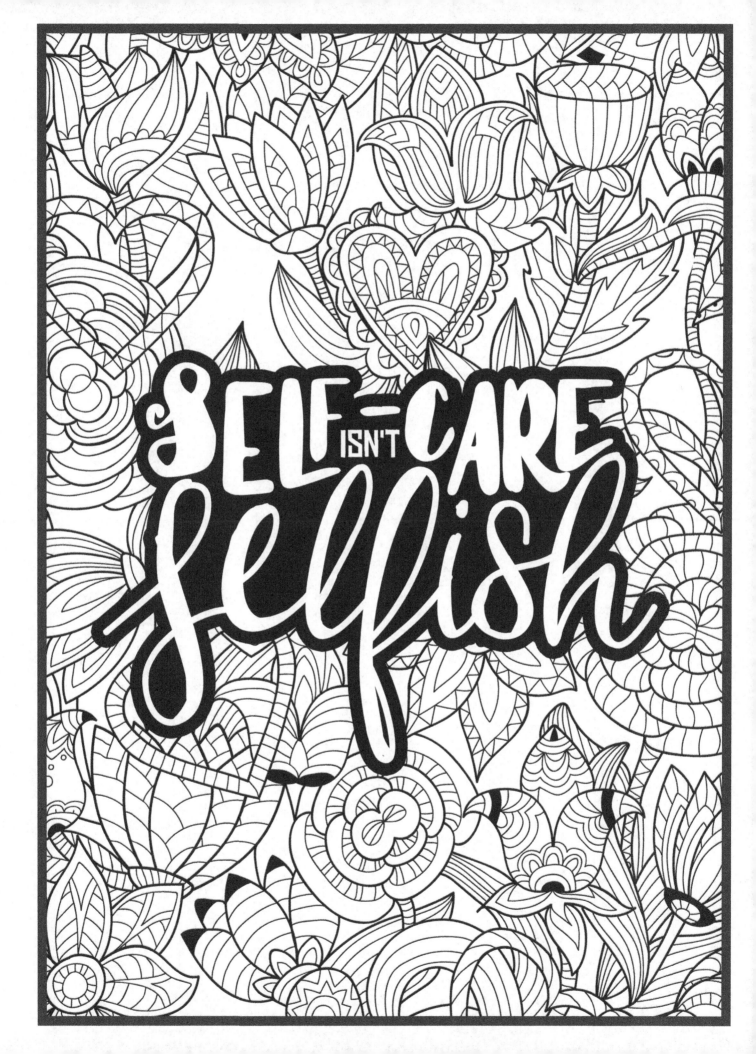

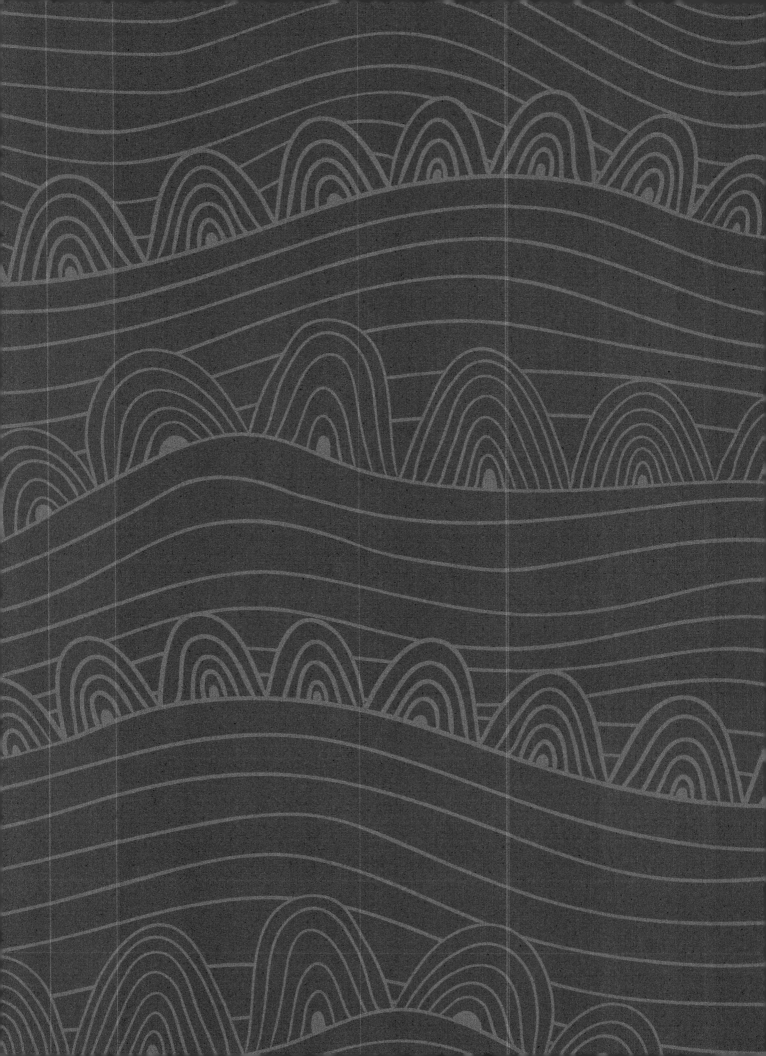

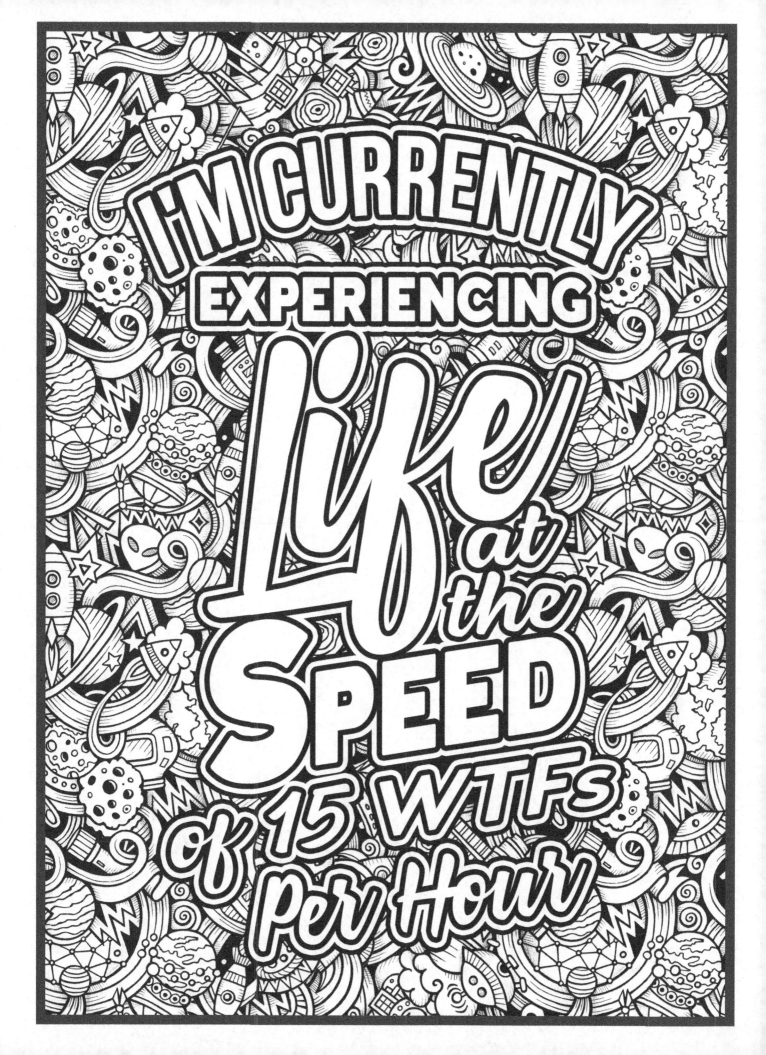

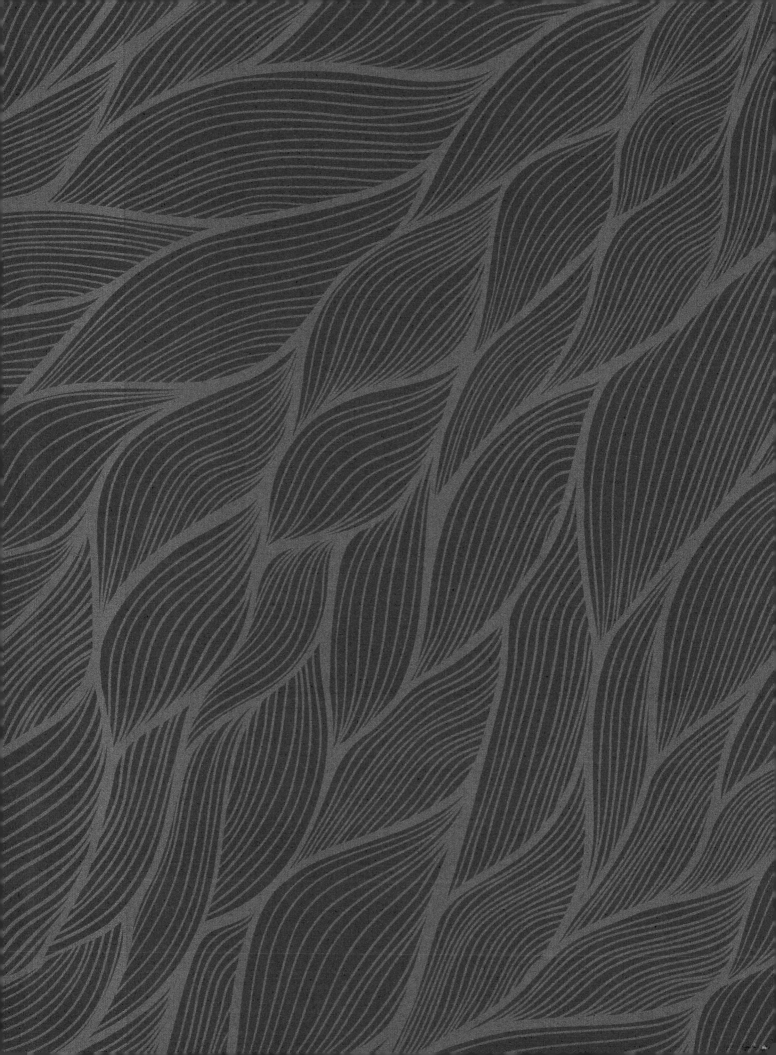

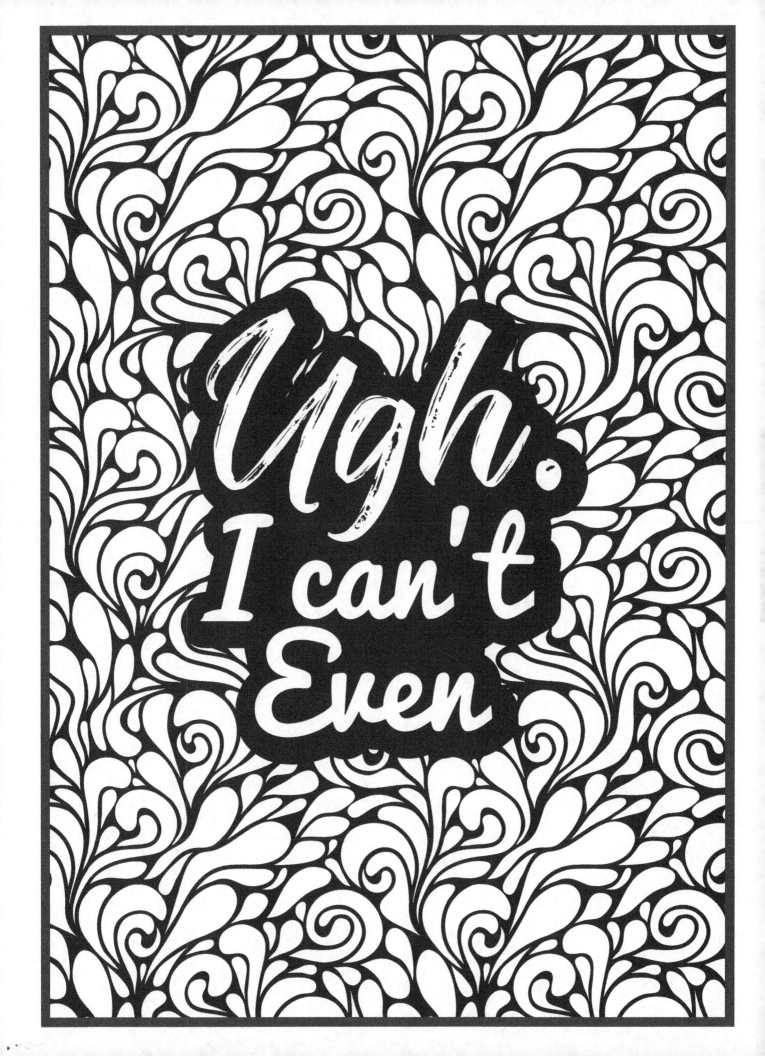

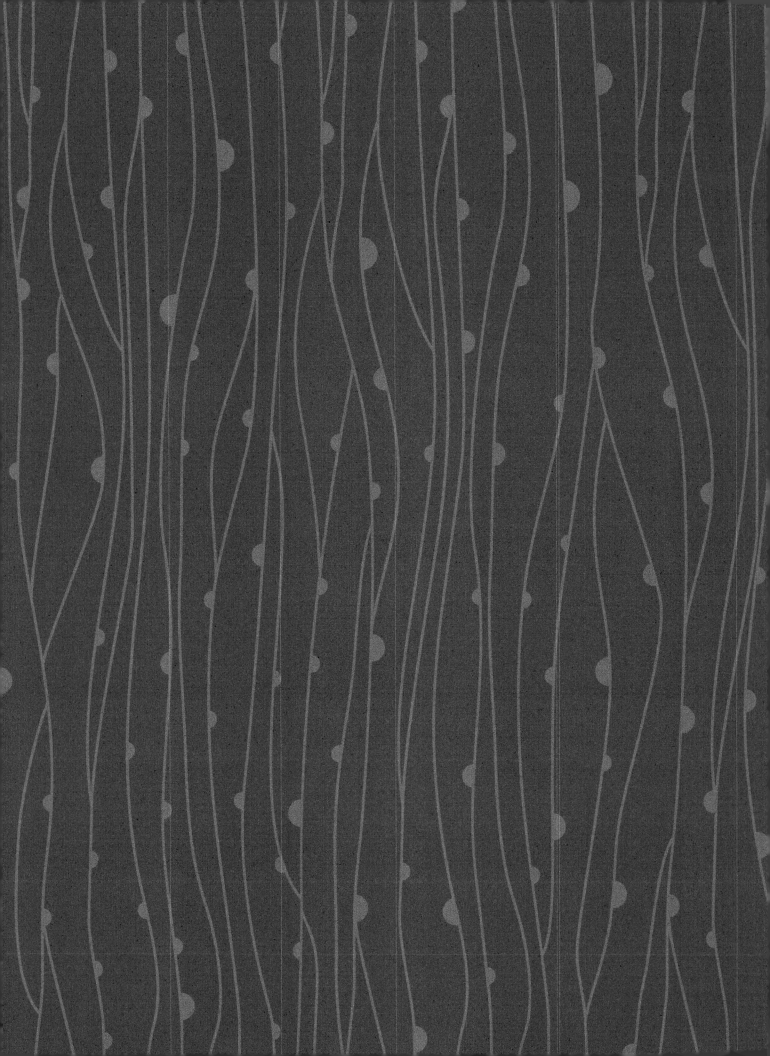

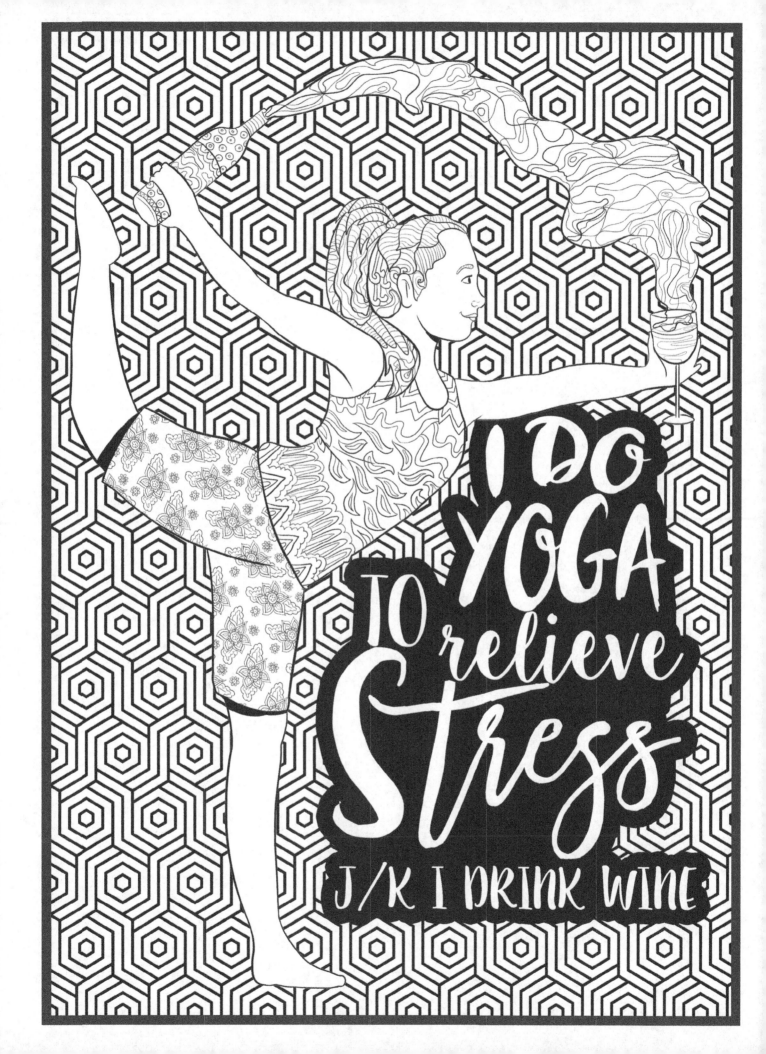

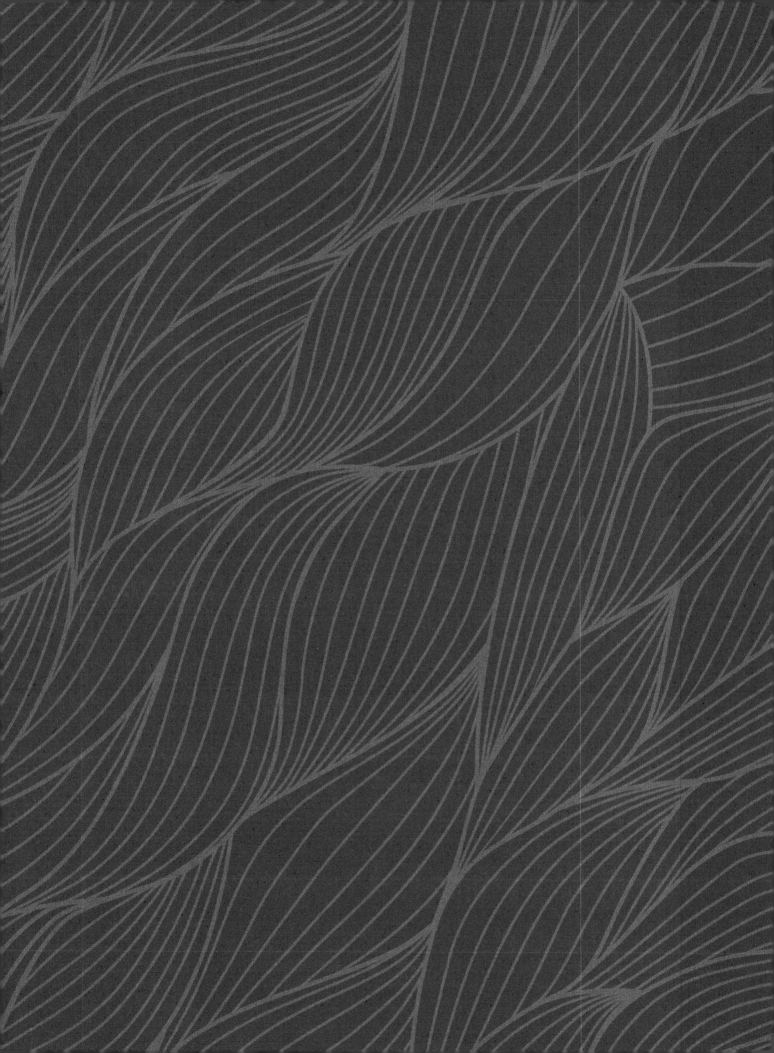

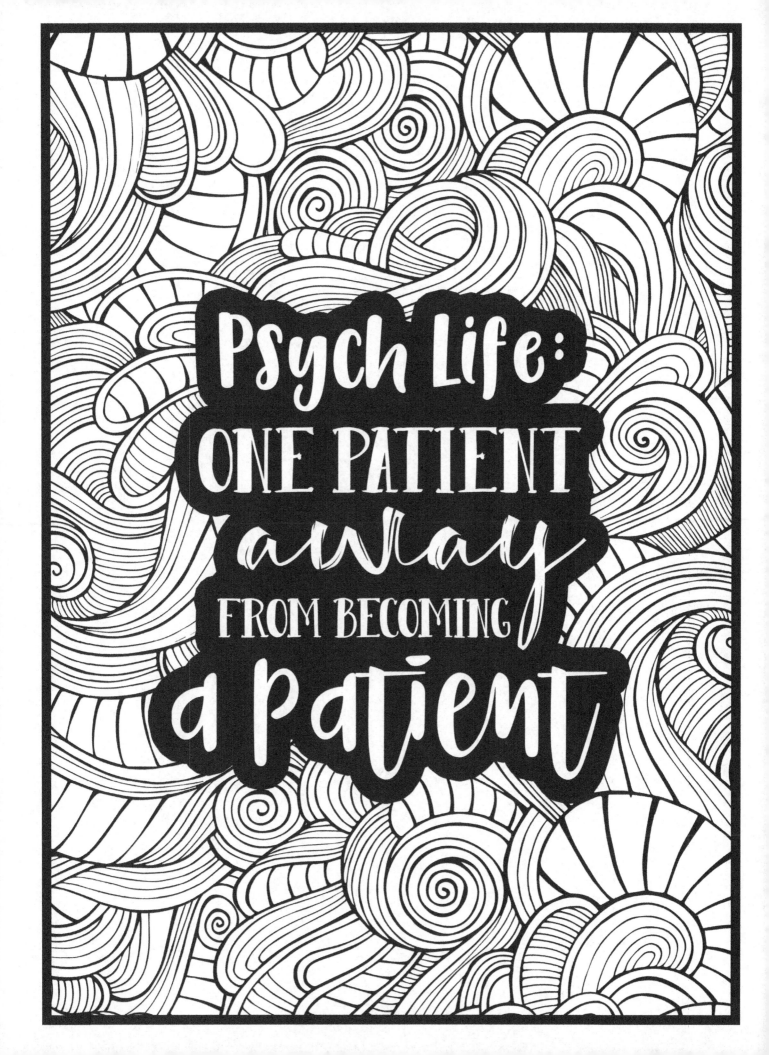

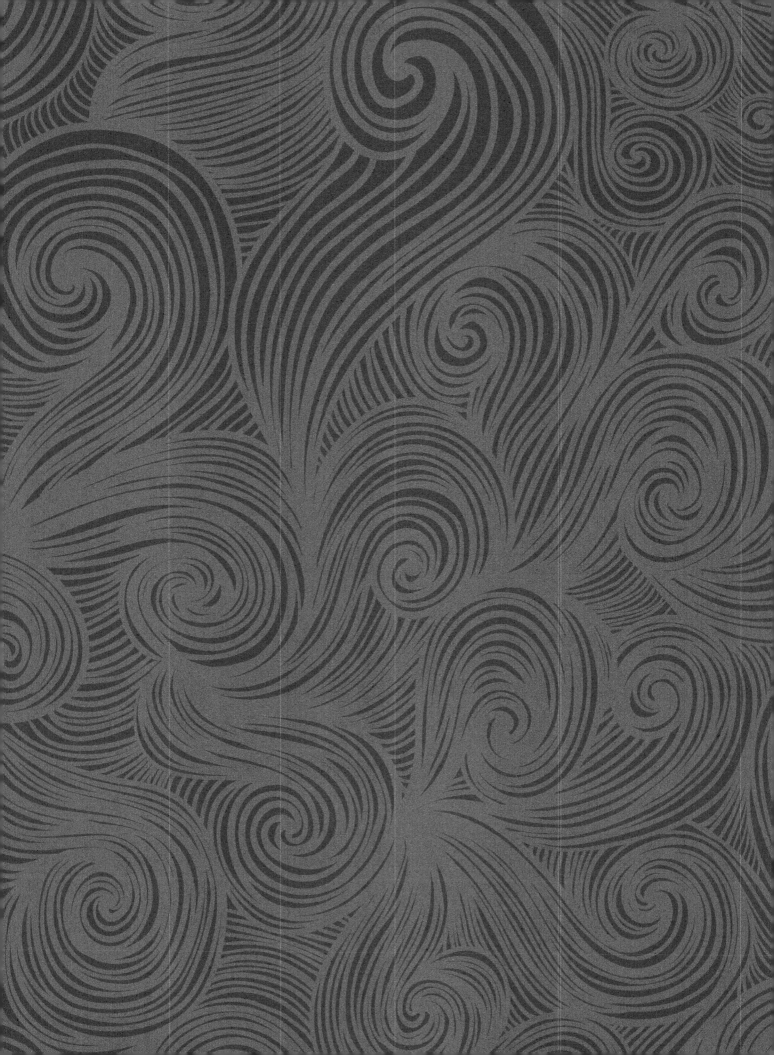

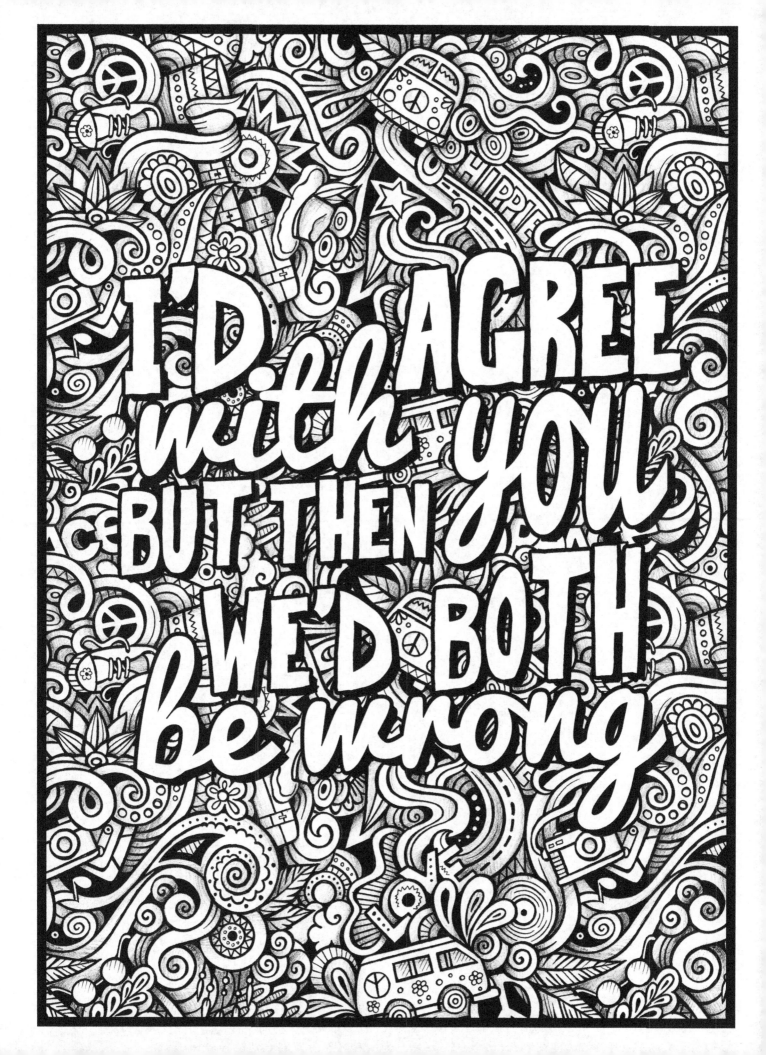

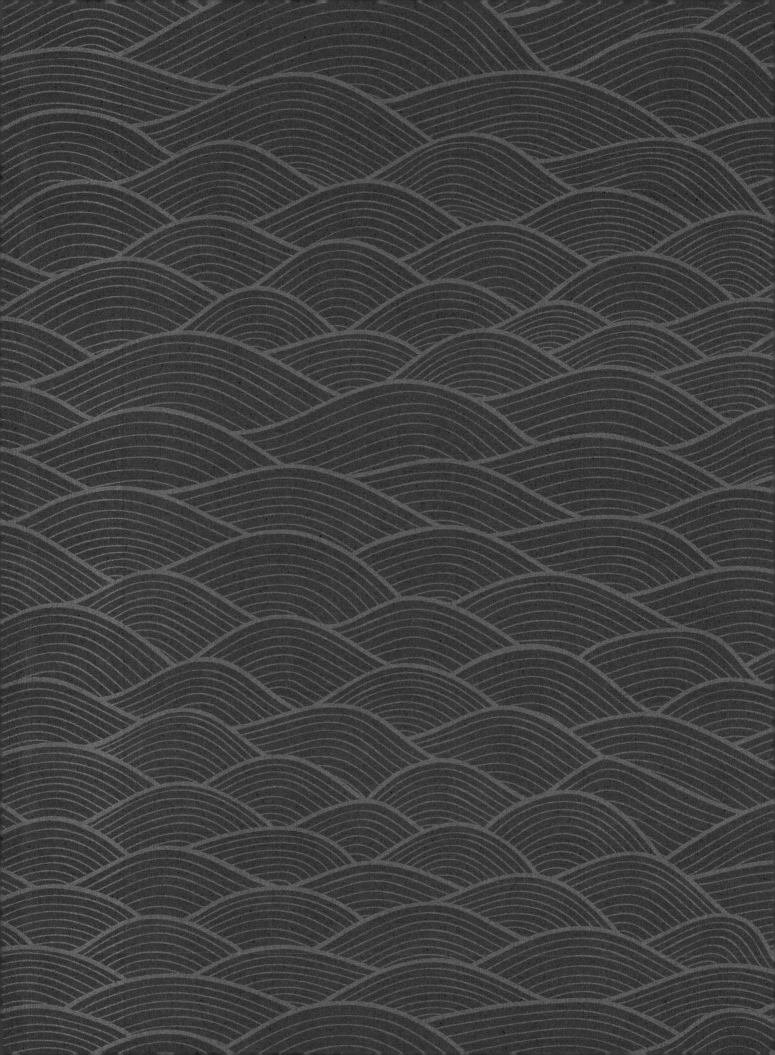

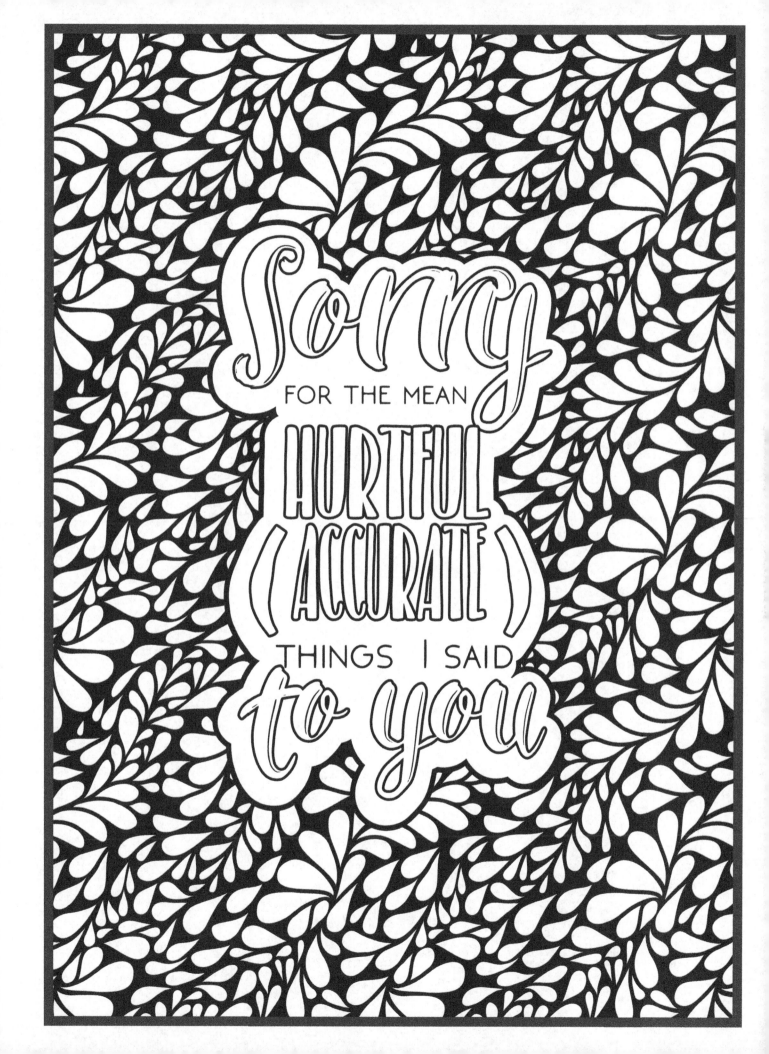

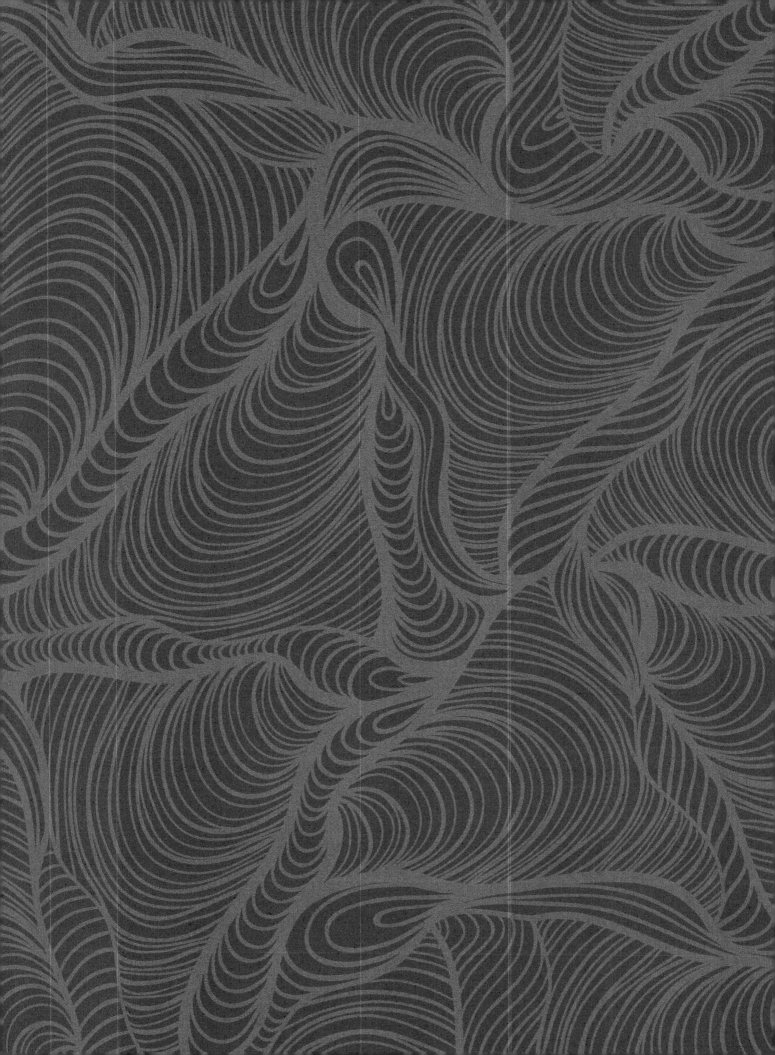

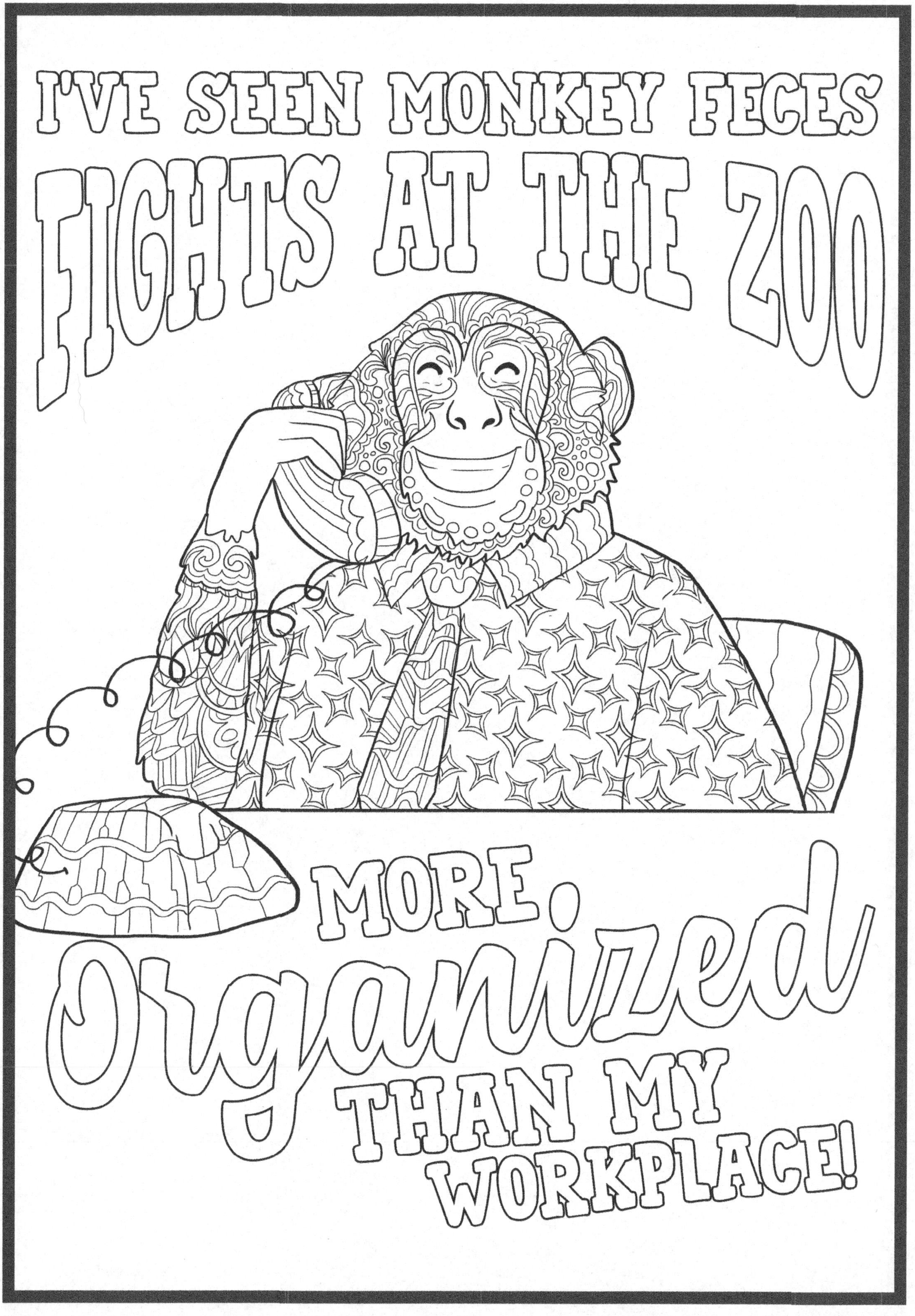
I'VE SEEN MONKEY FECES
FIGHTS AT THE ZOO
MORE
Organized
THAN MY
WORKPLACE!

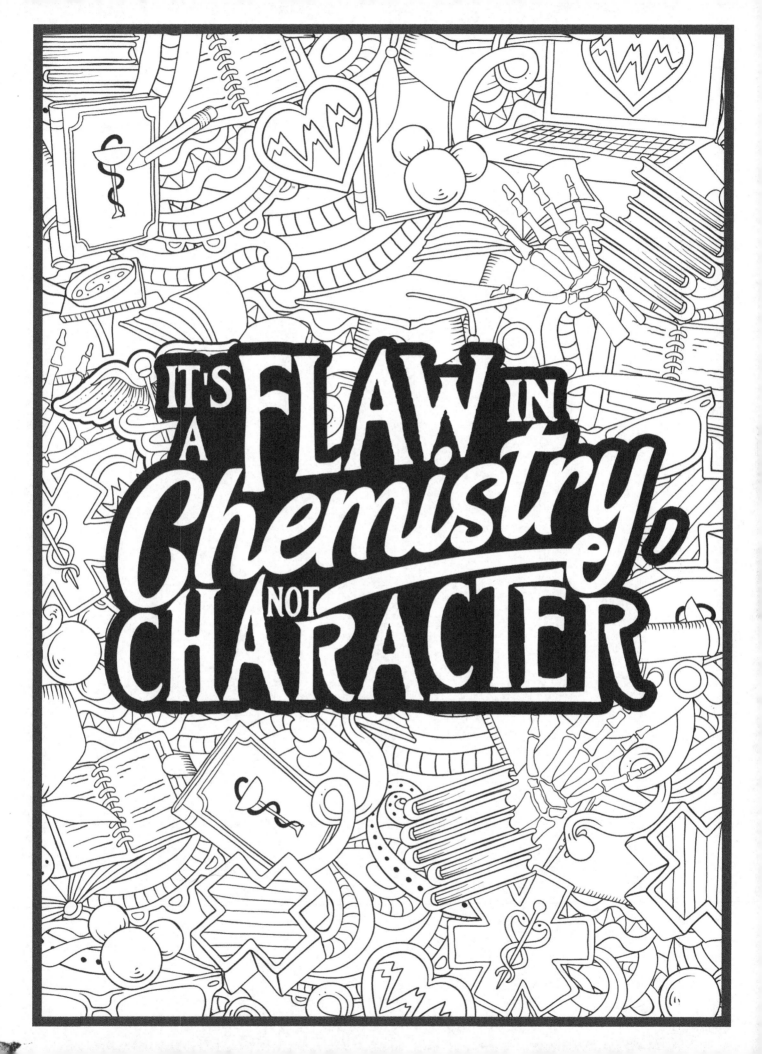

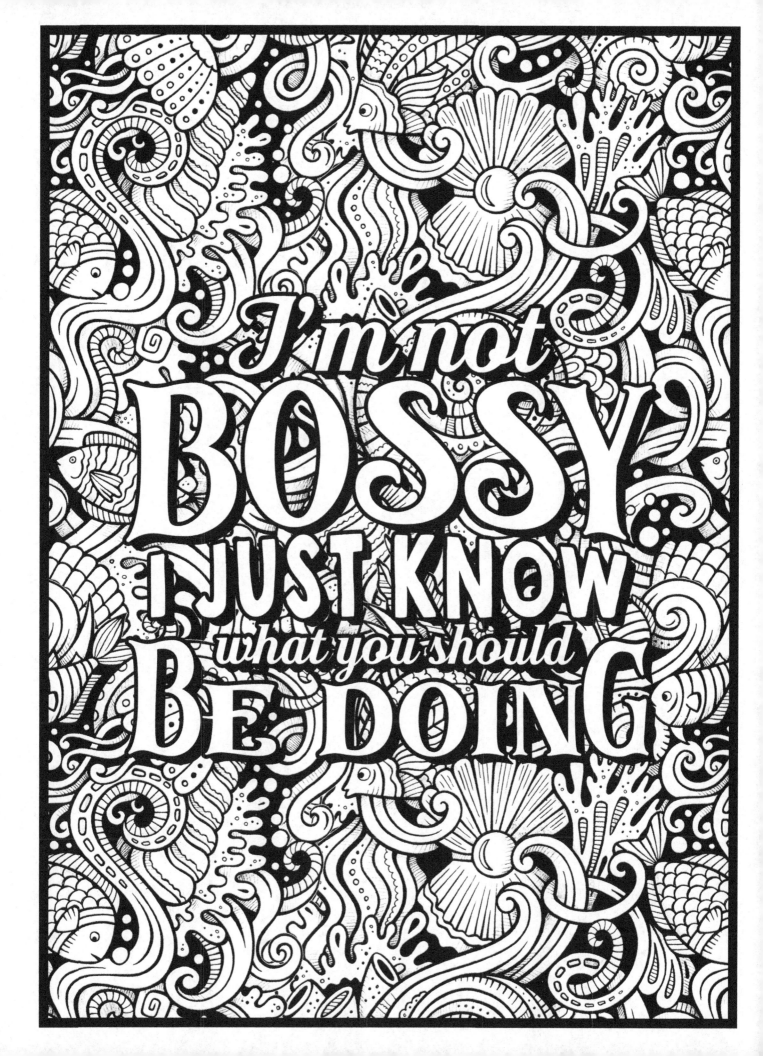

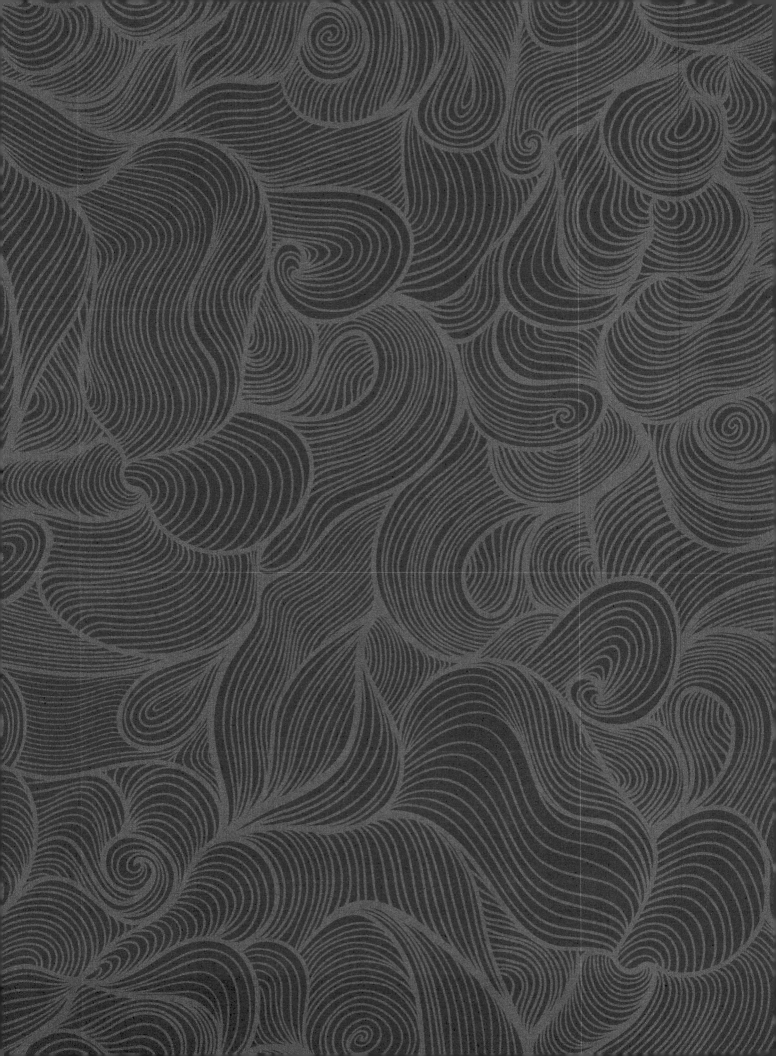

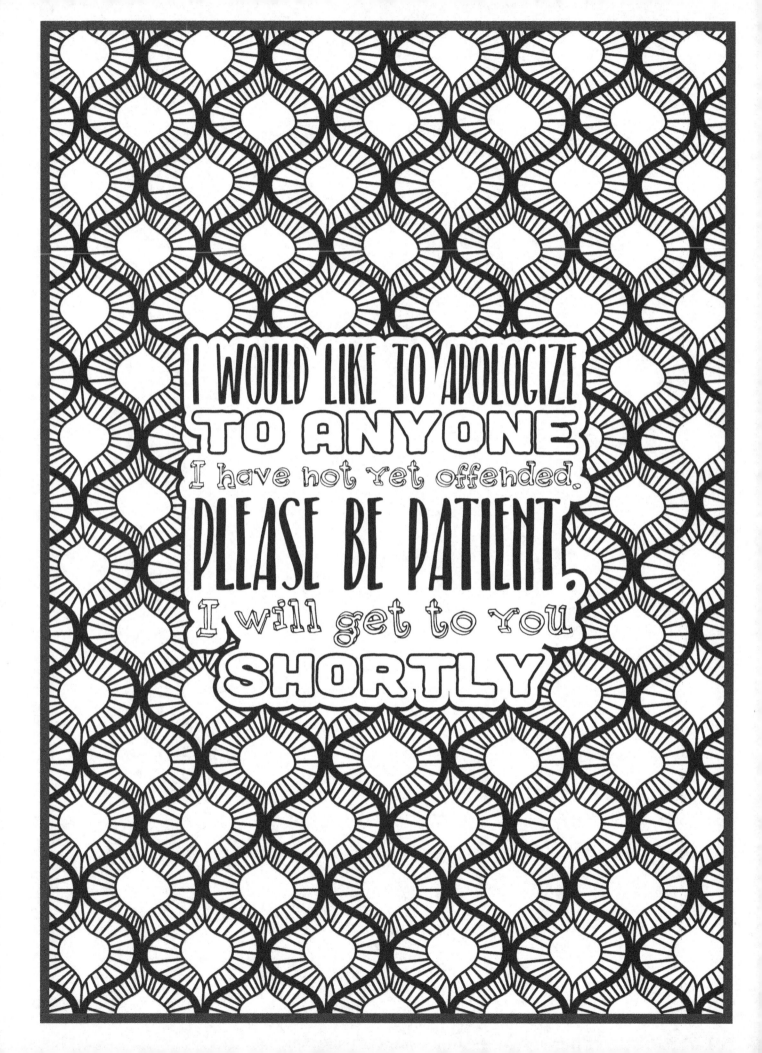

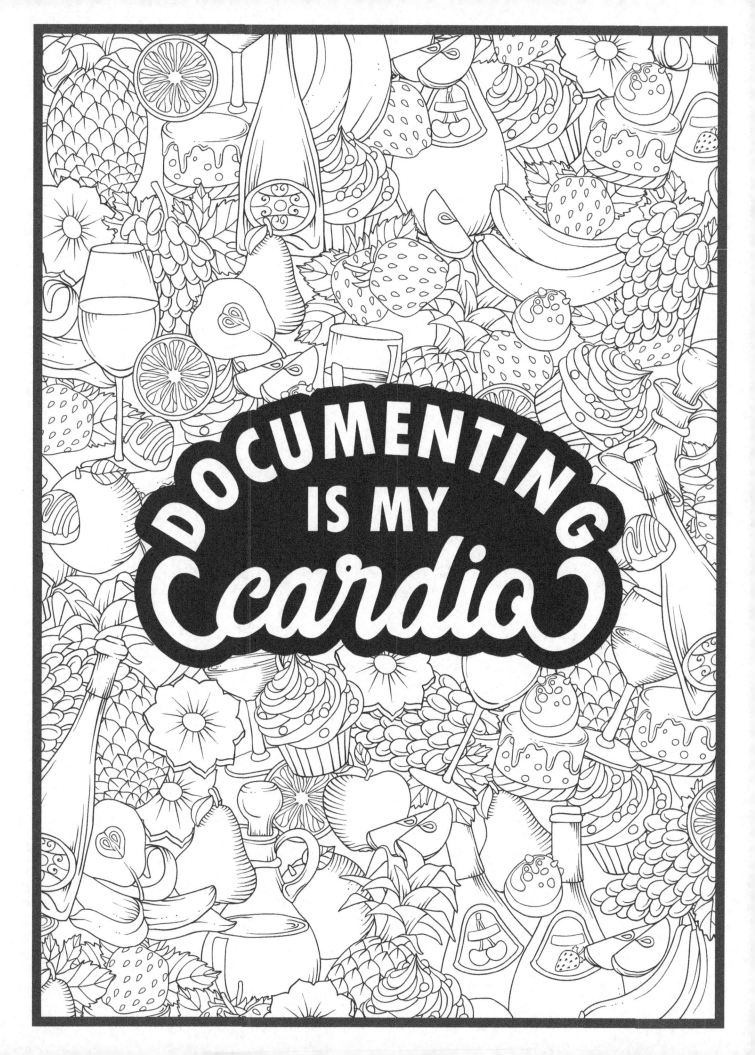

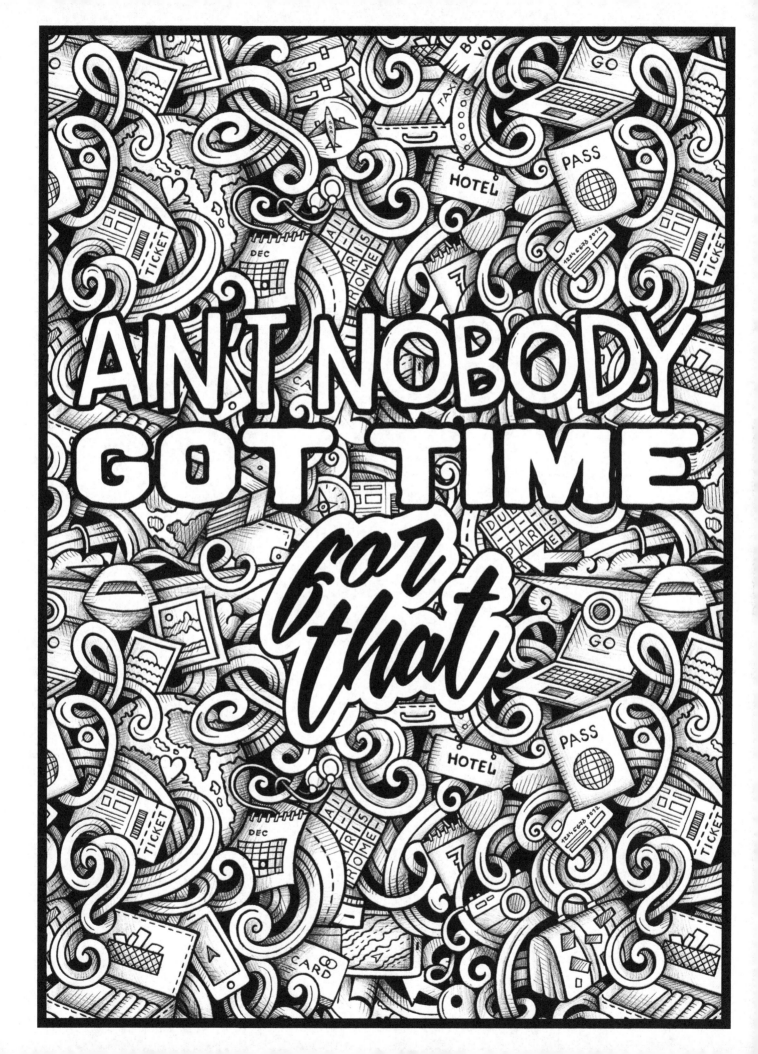

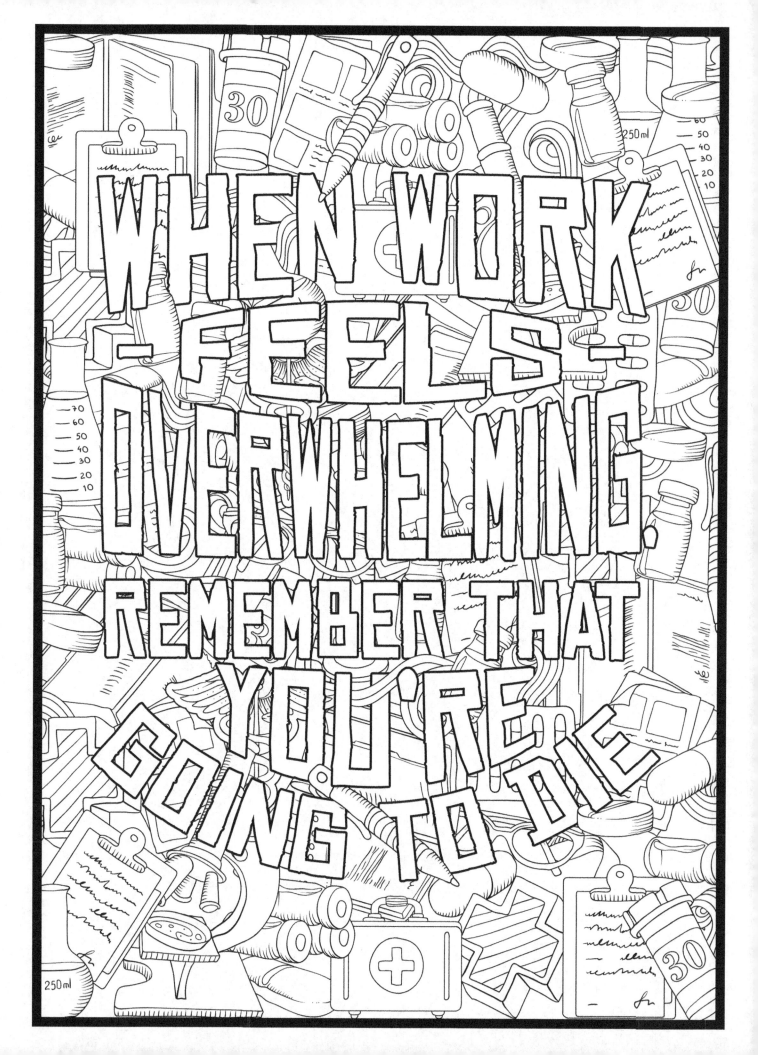

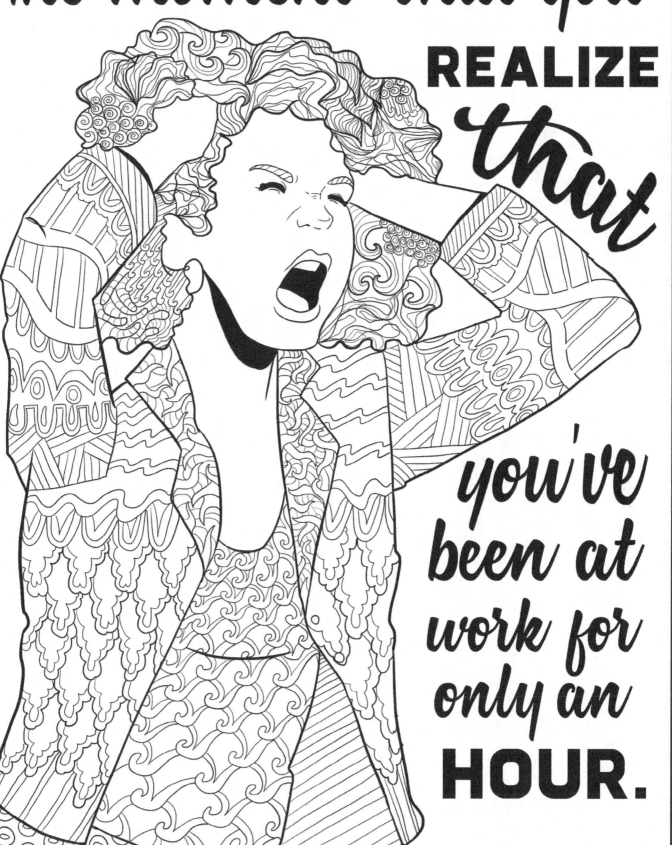

The moment that you REALIZE that you've been at work for only an HOUR.

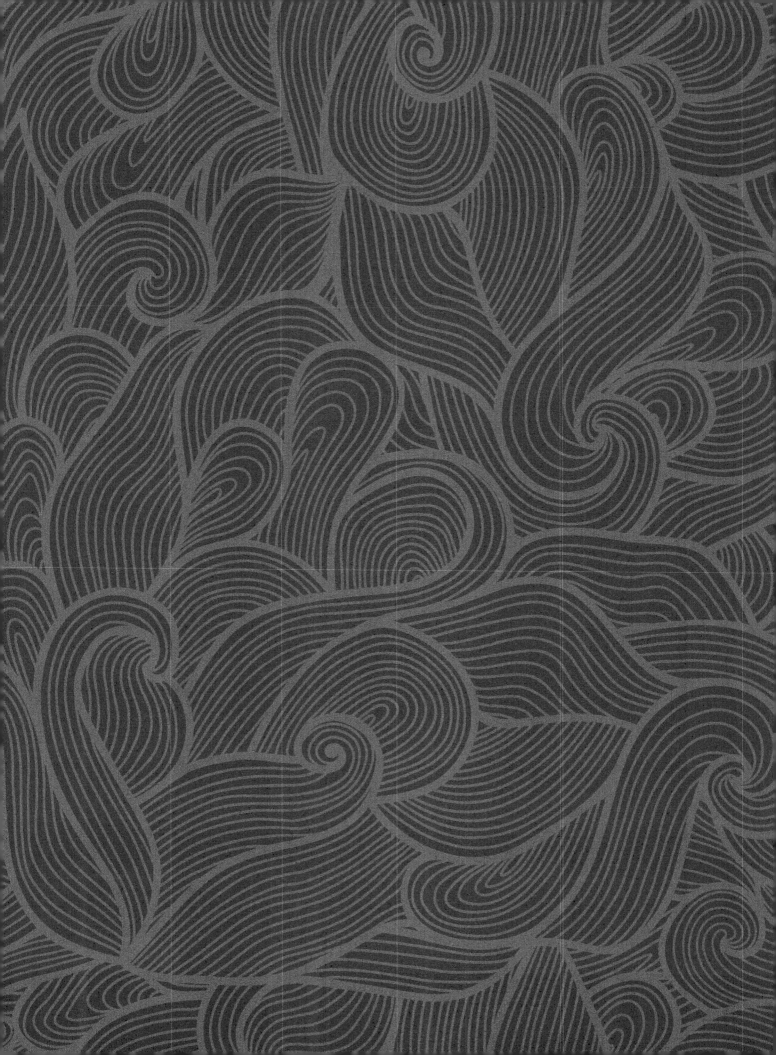

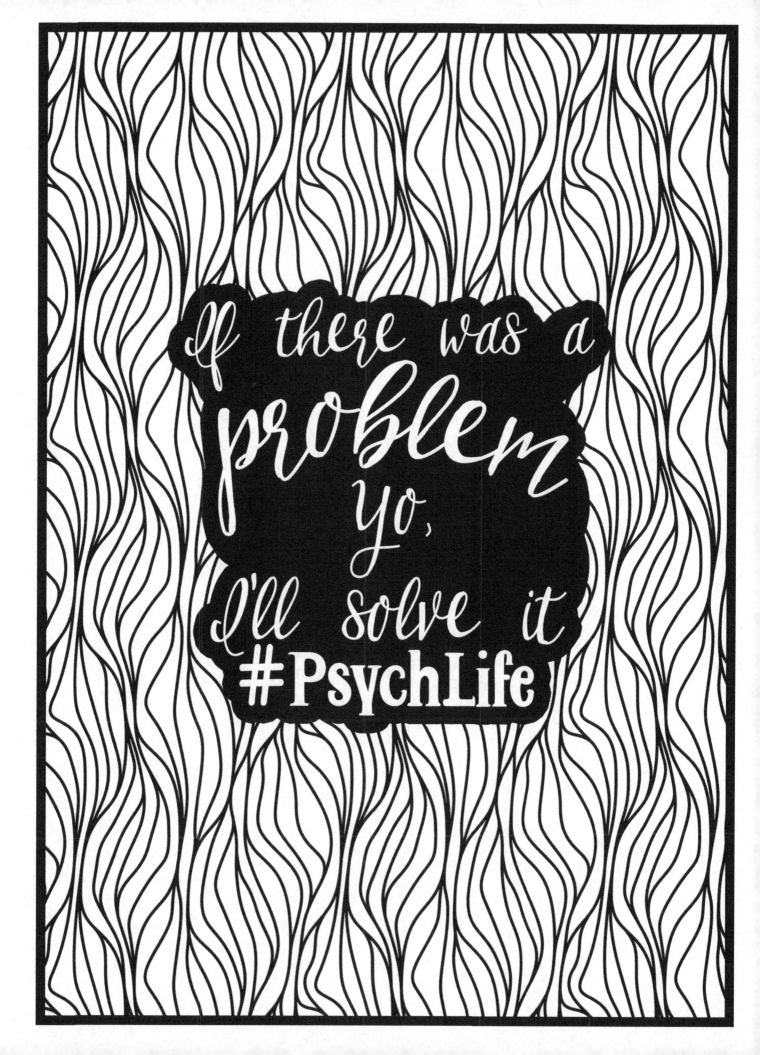

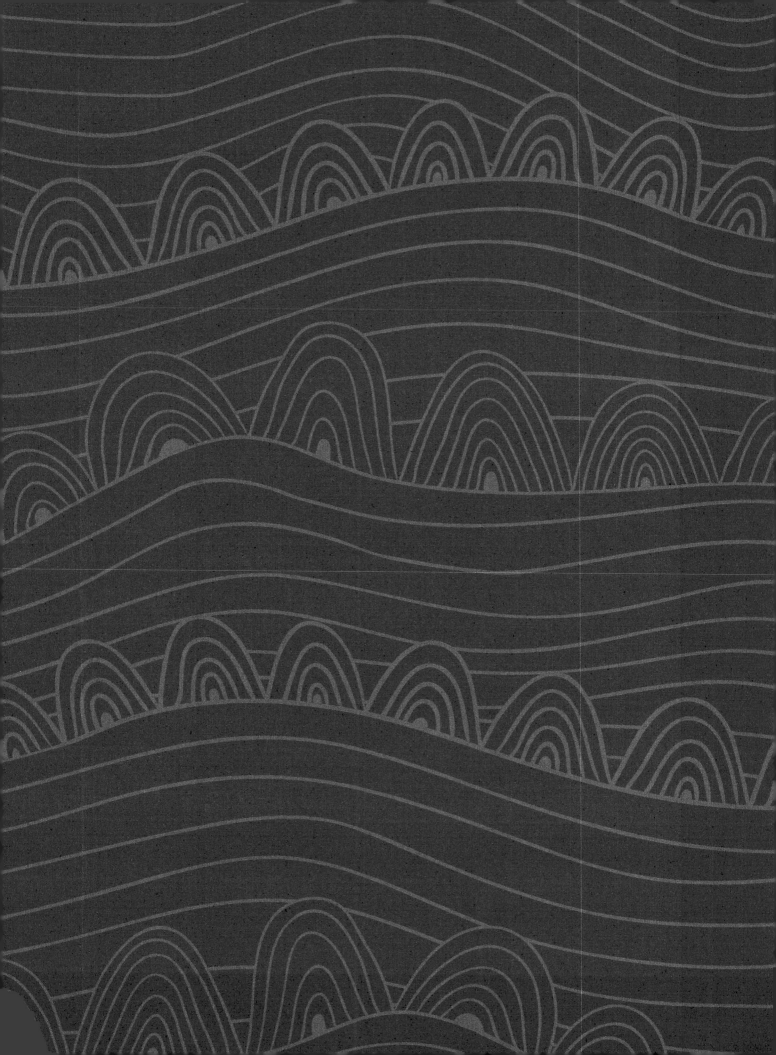

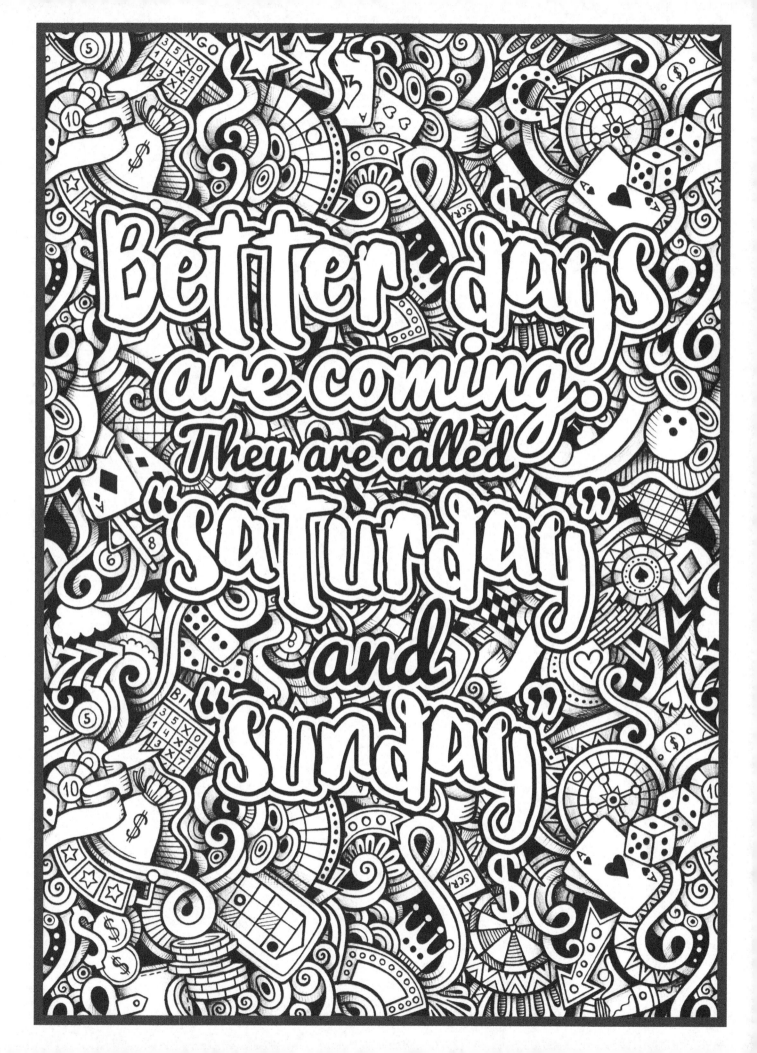

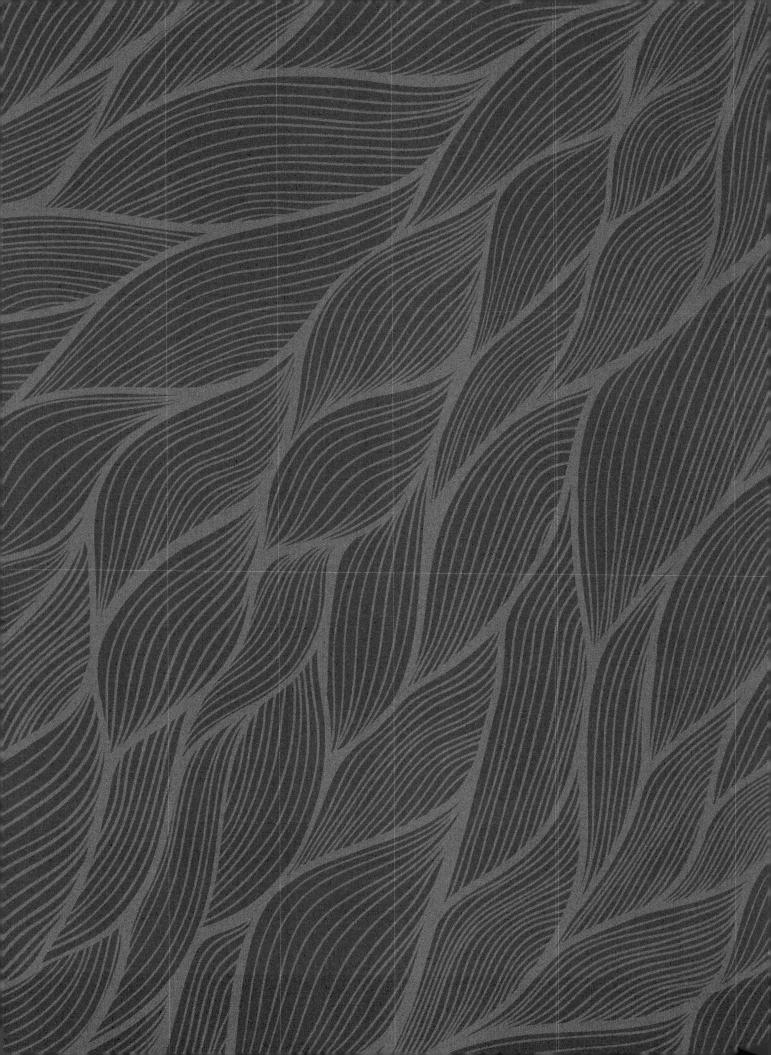

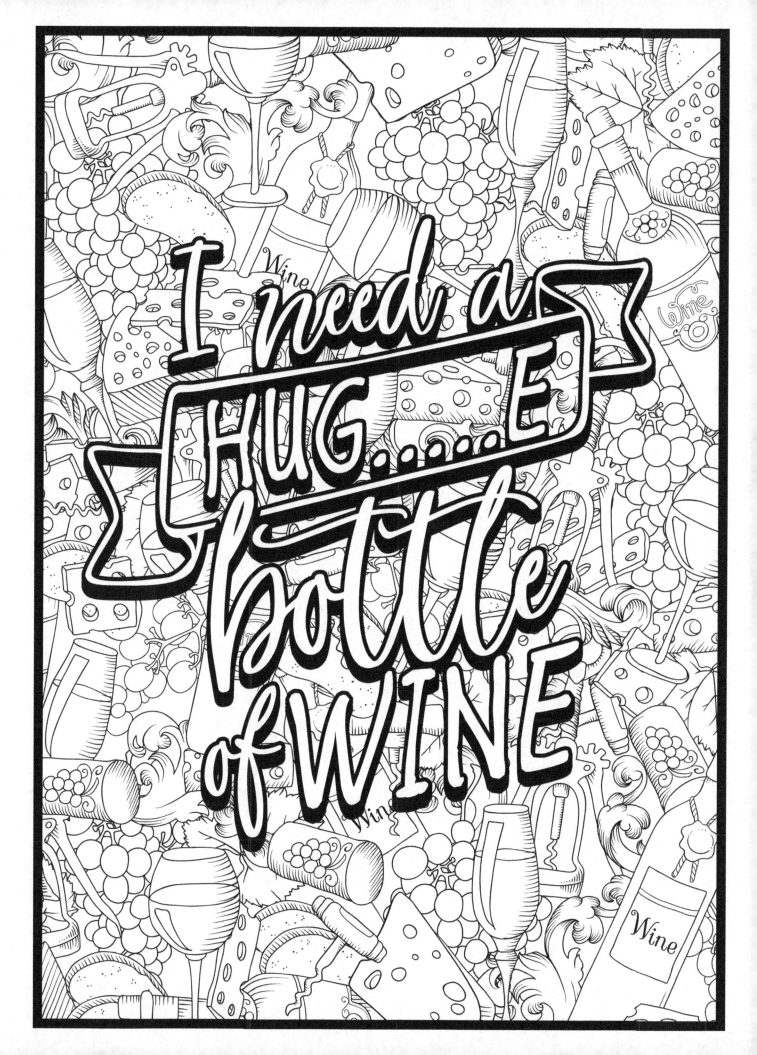

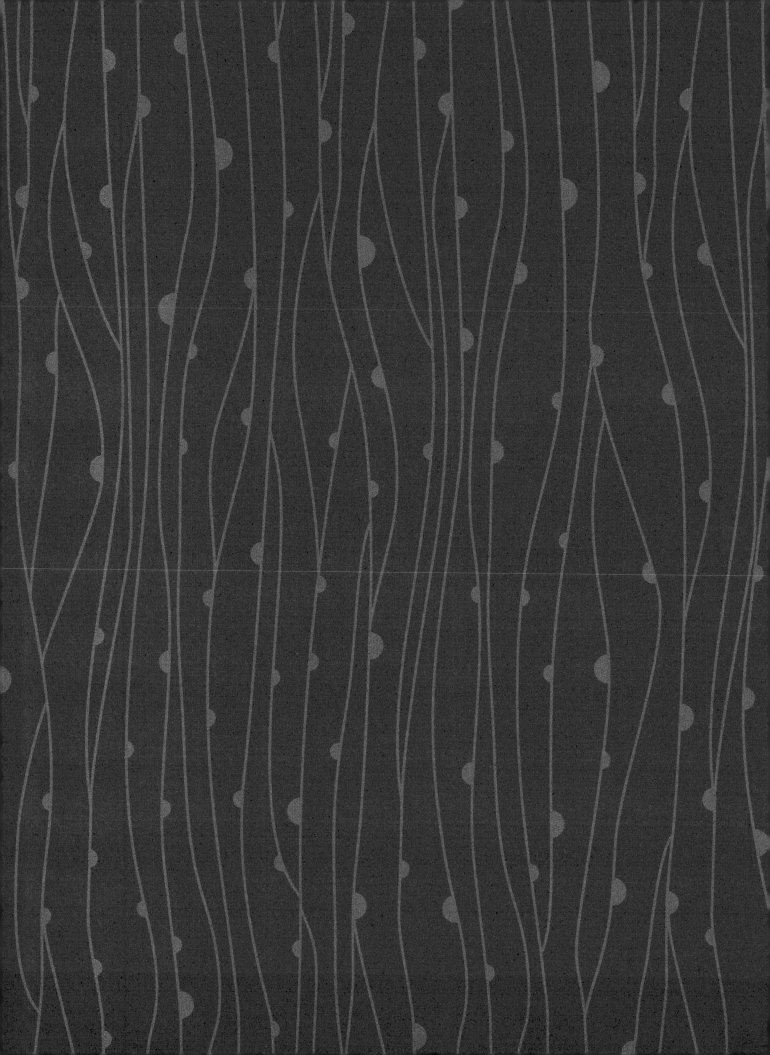

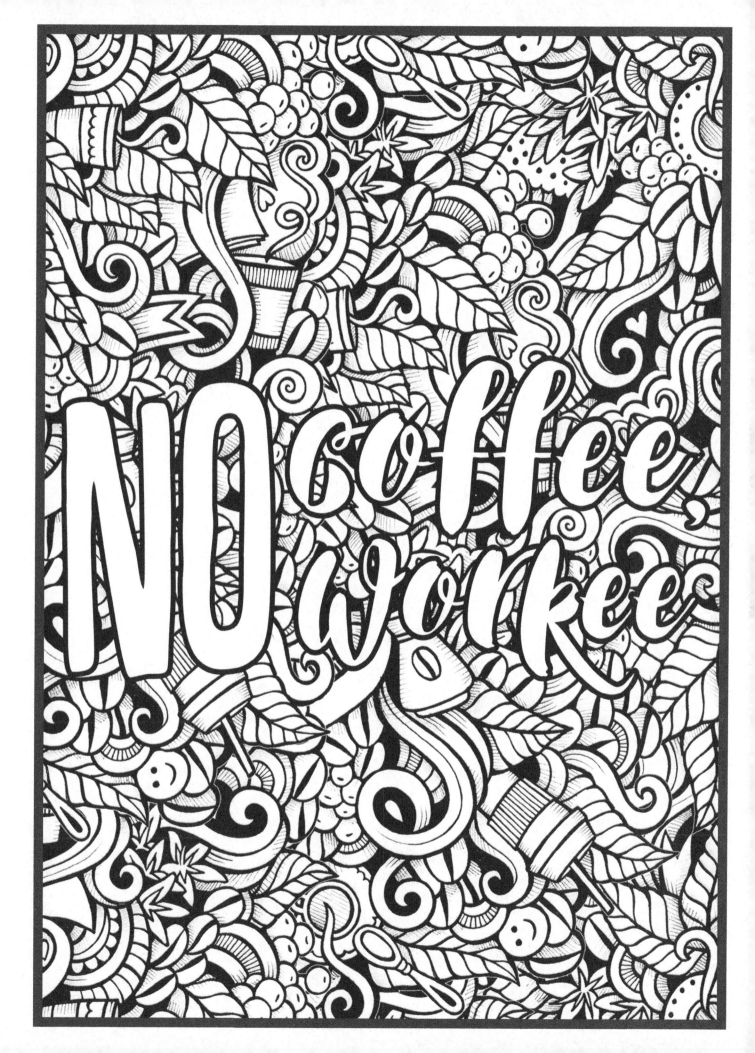

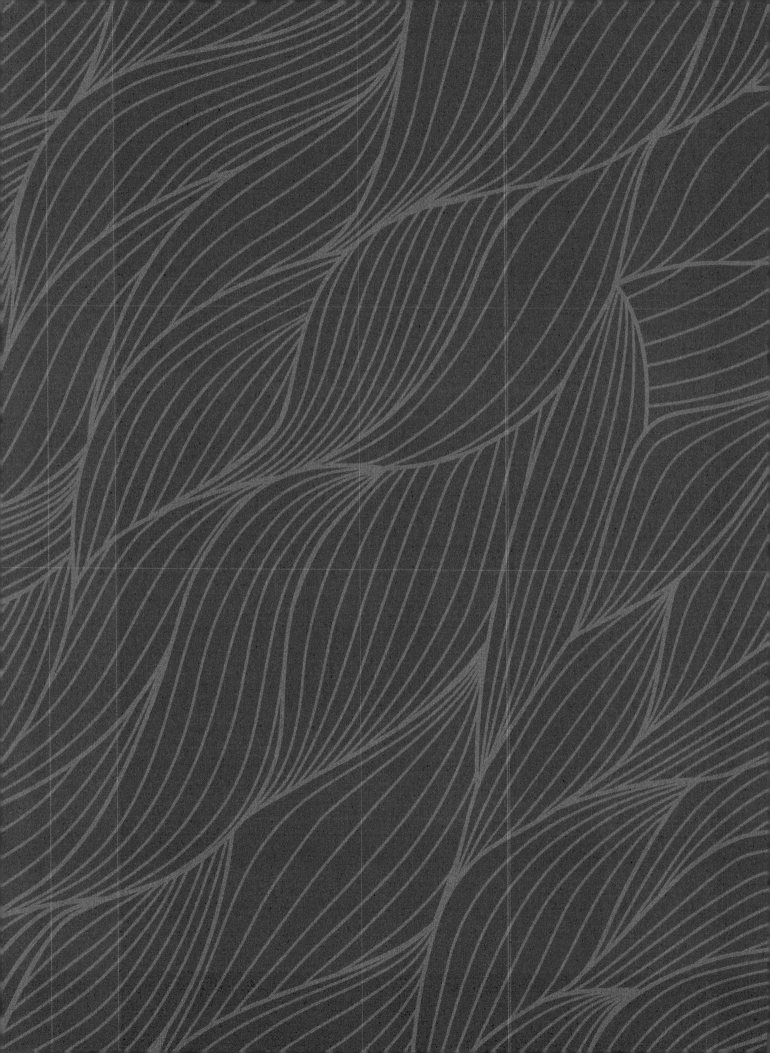

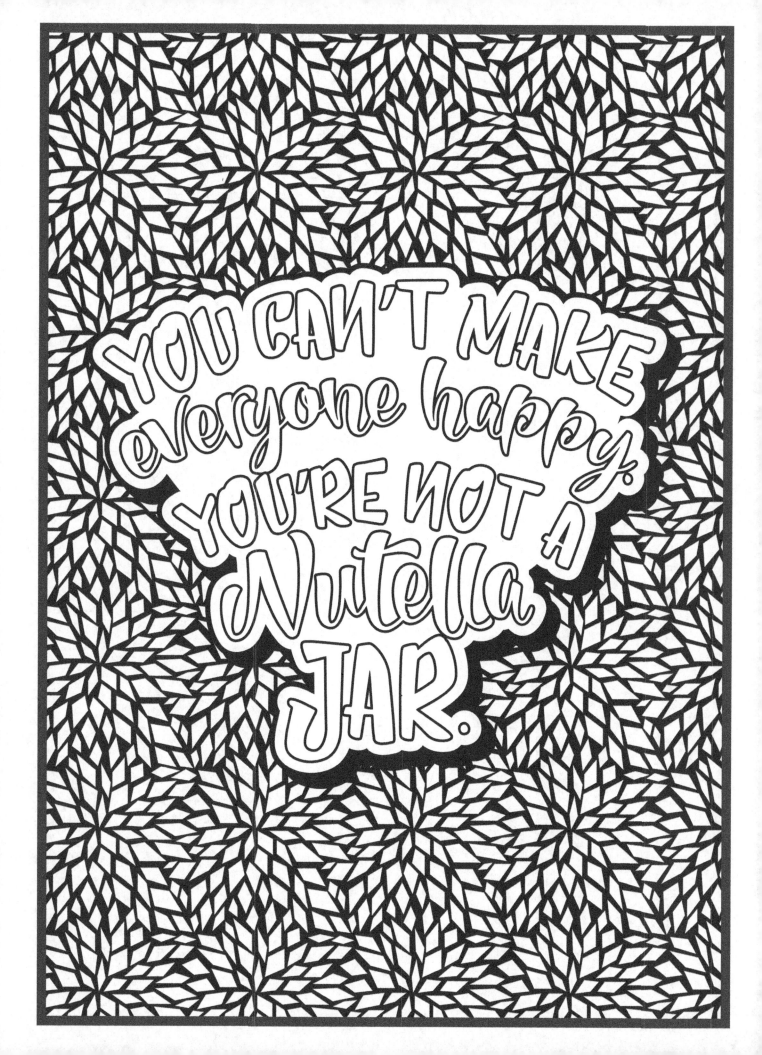

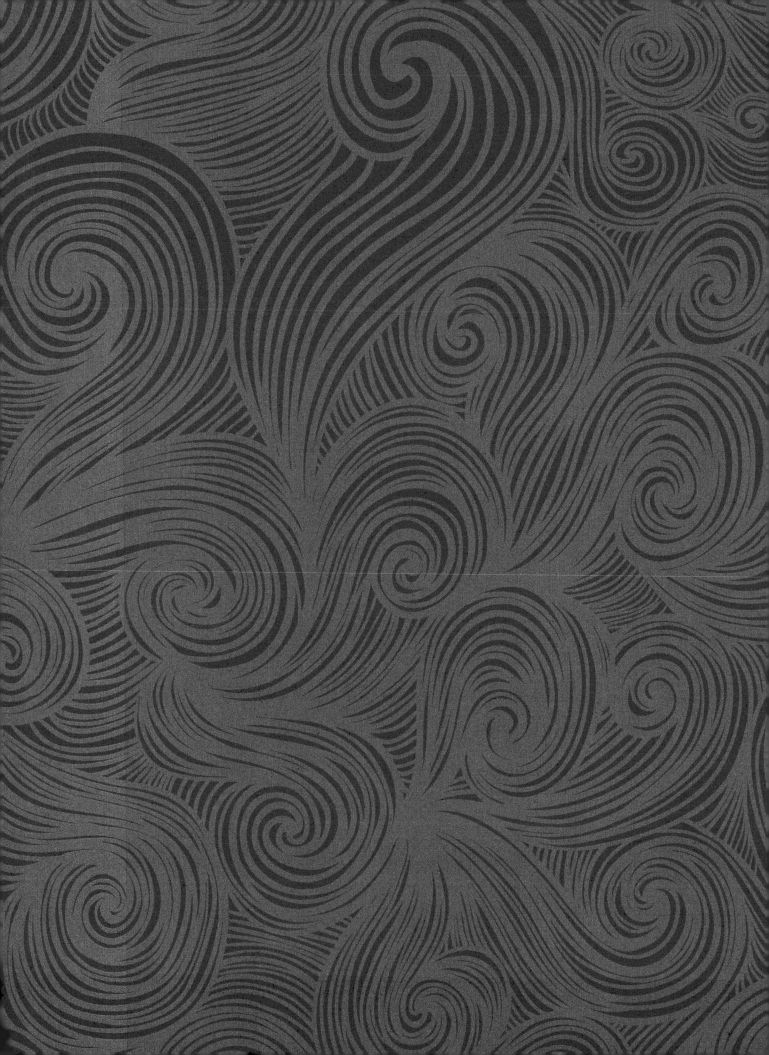

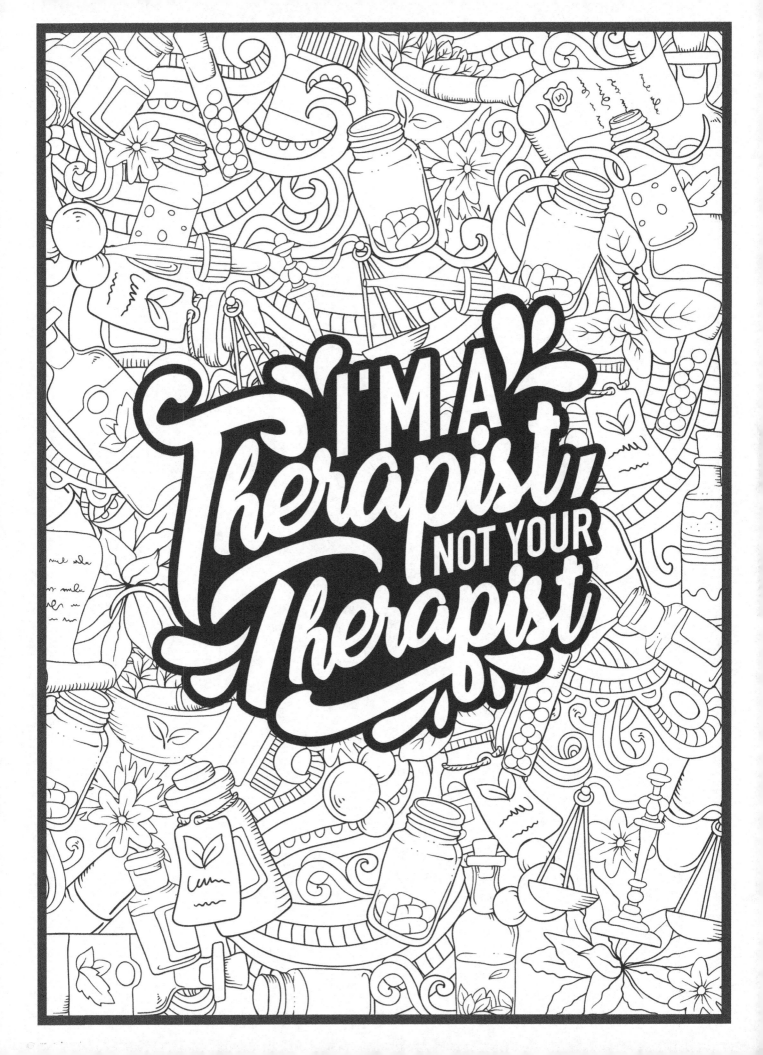

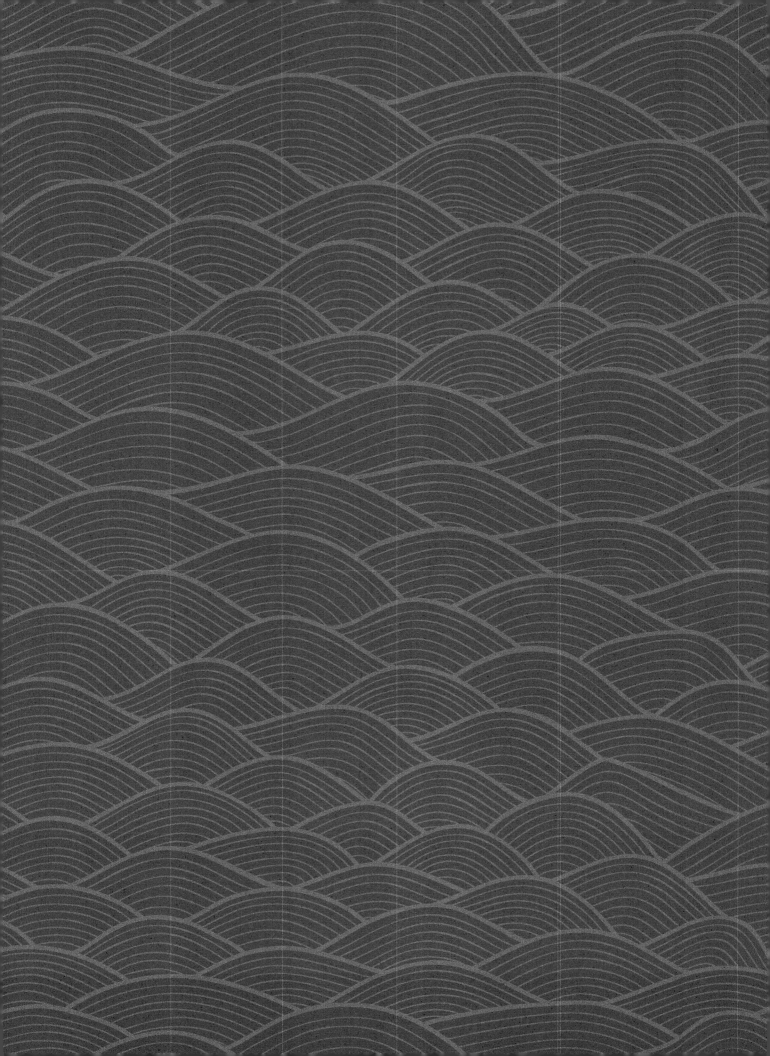

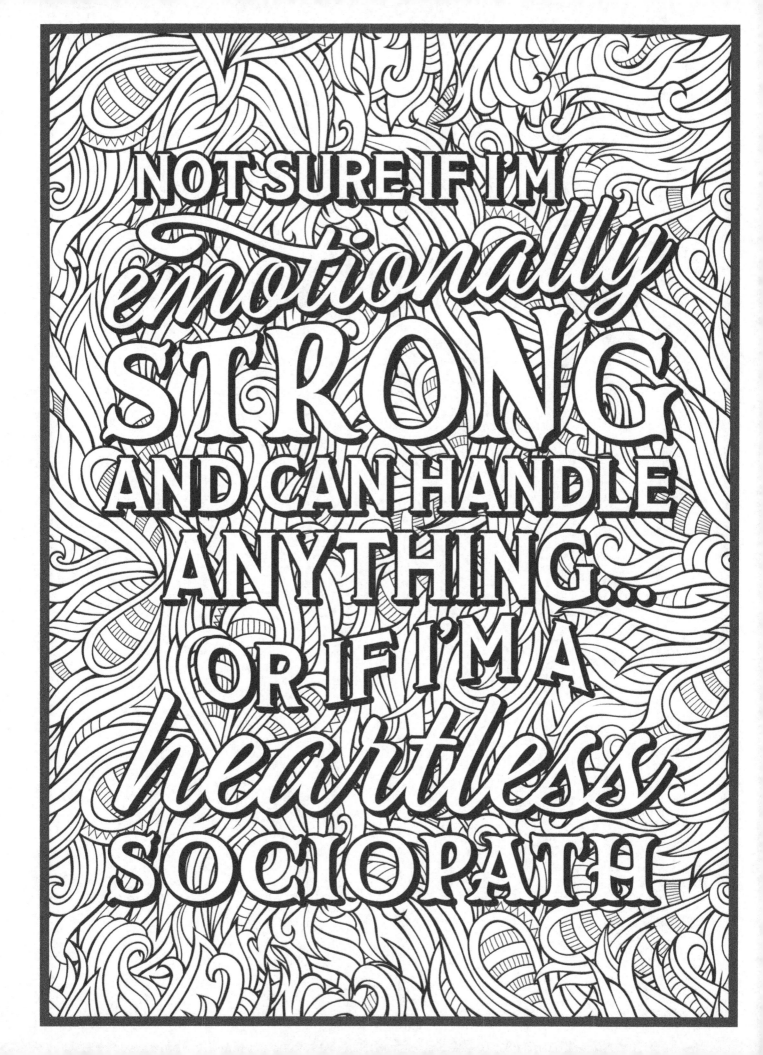

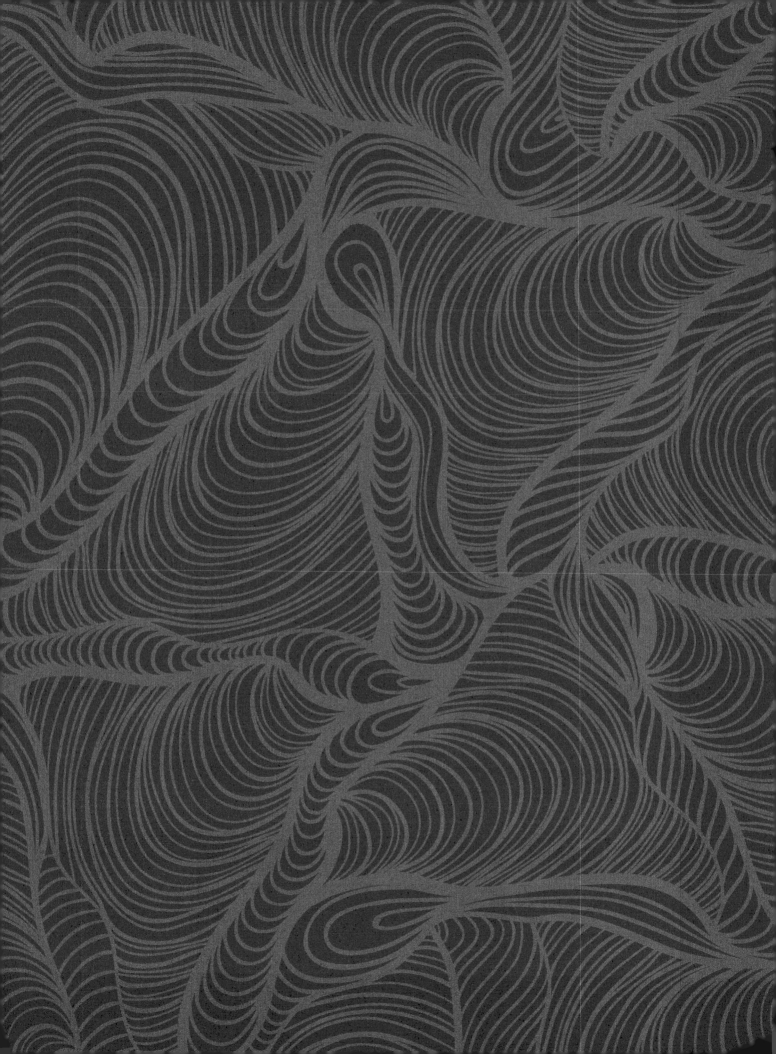

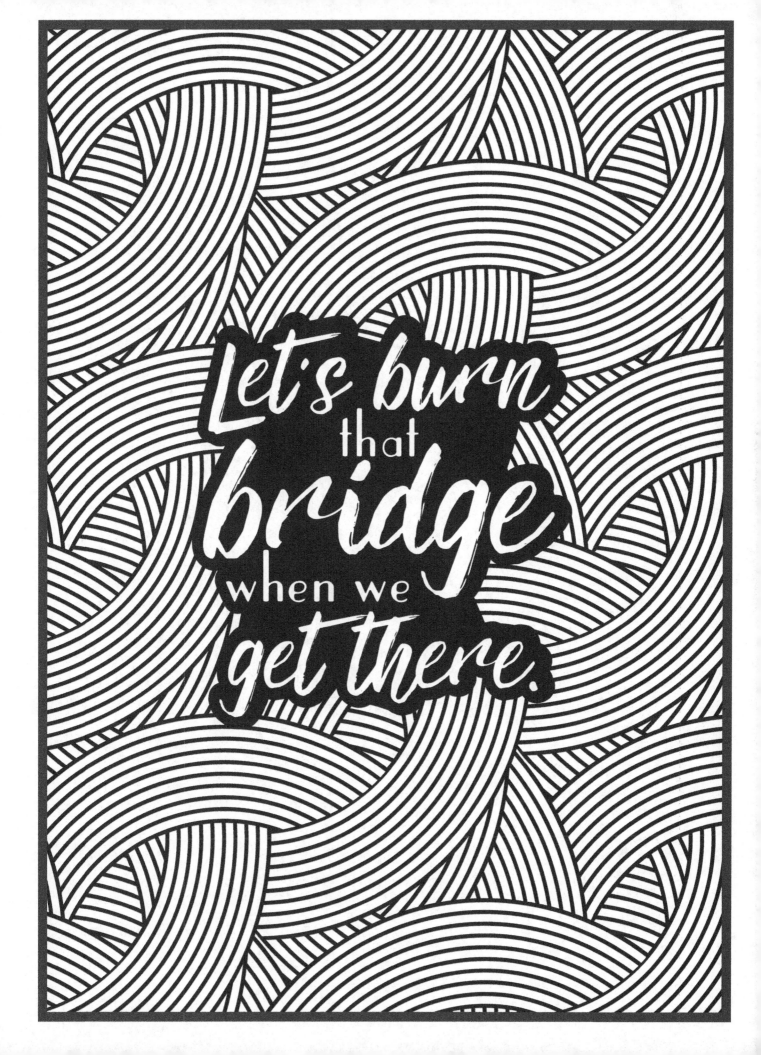

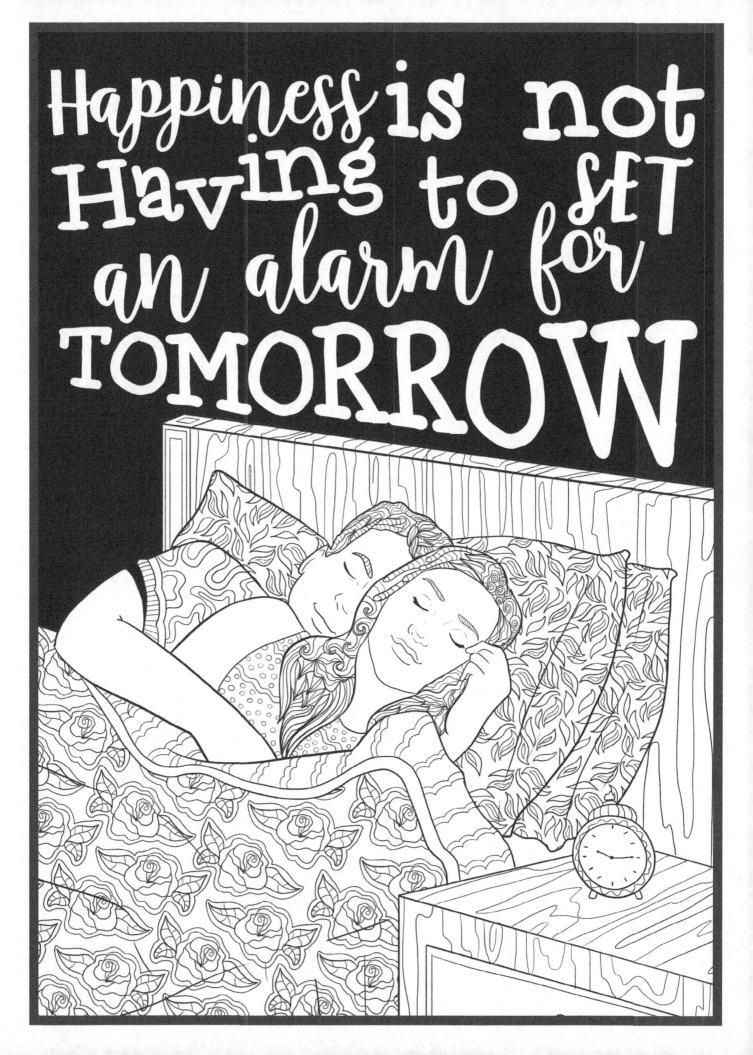

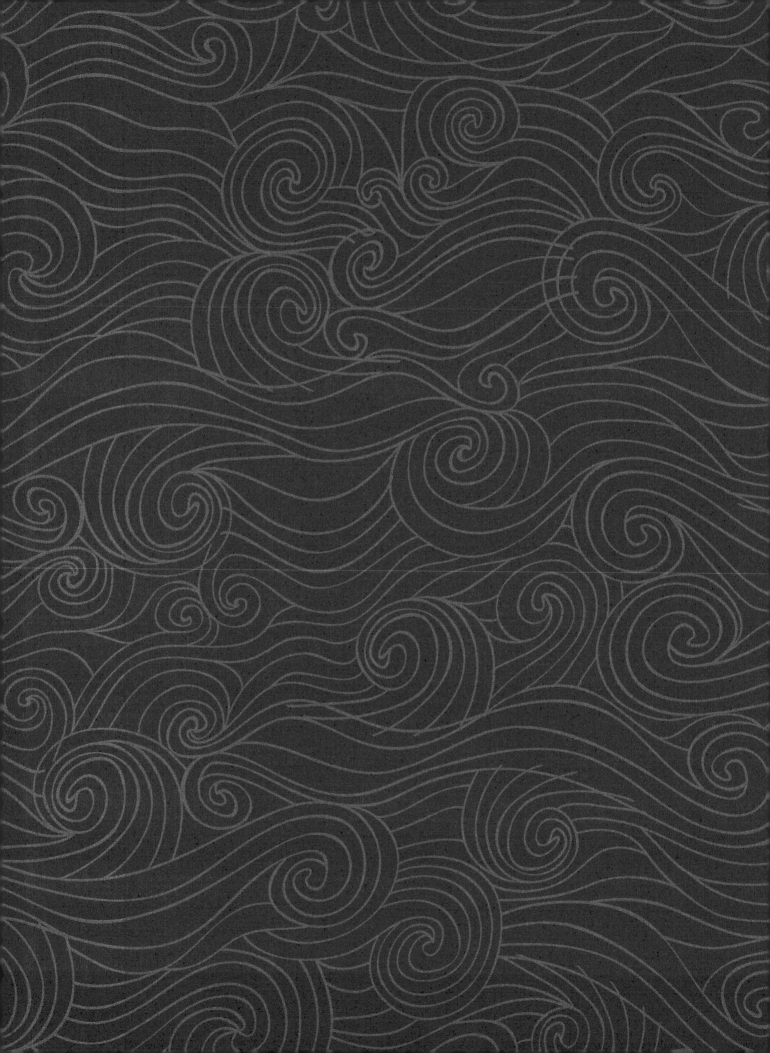

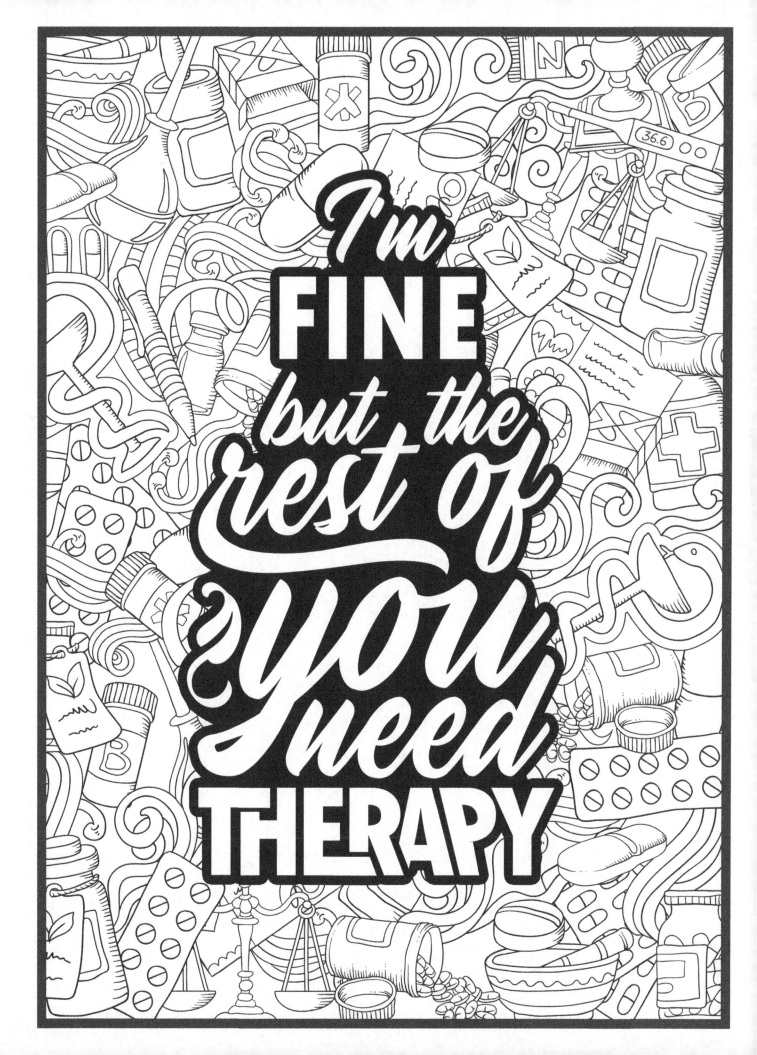

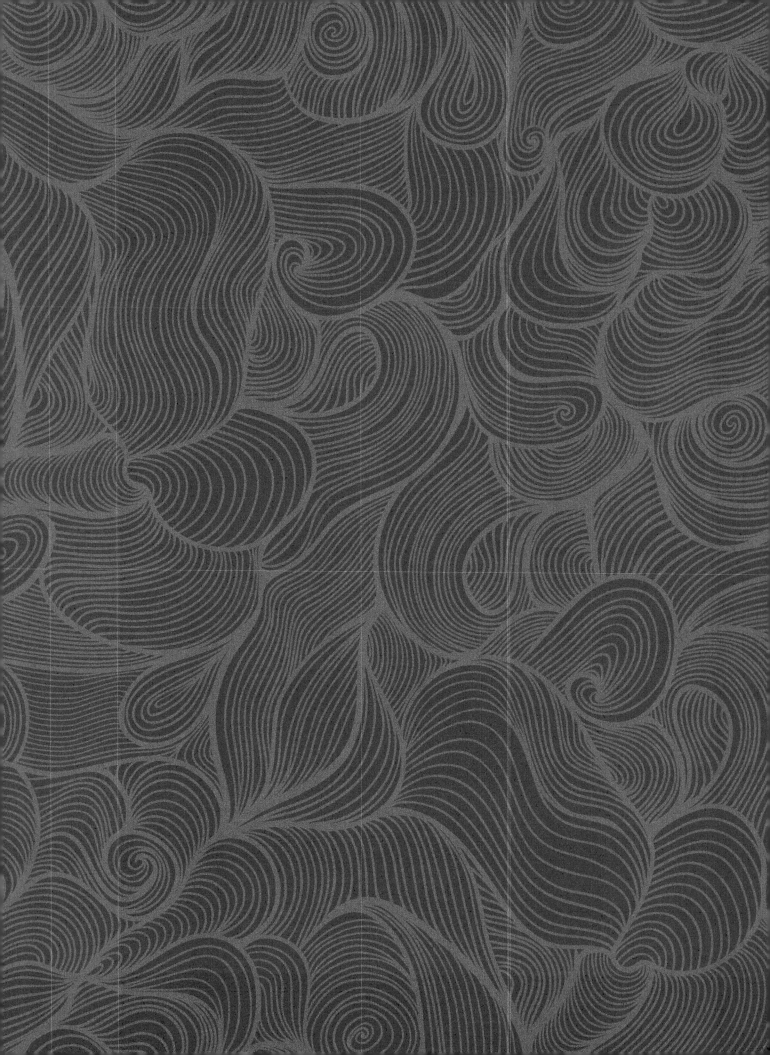

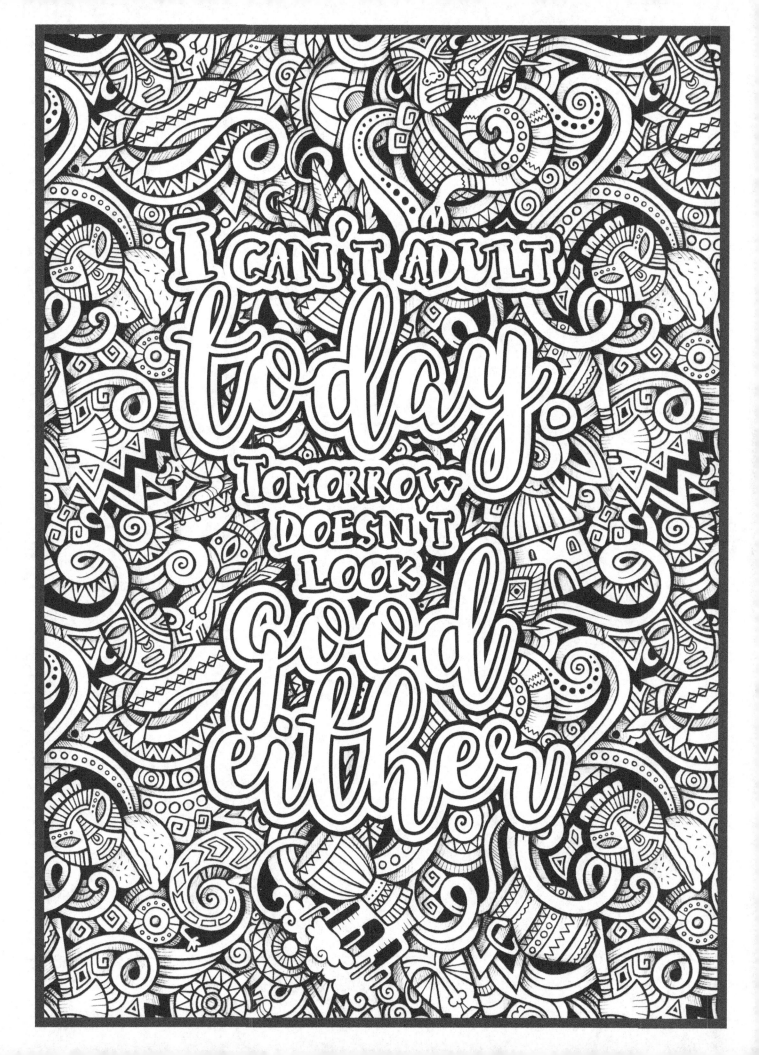

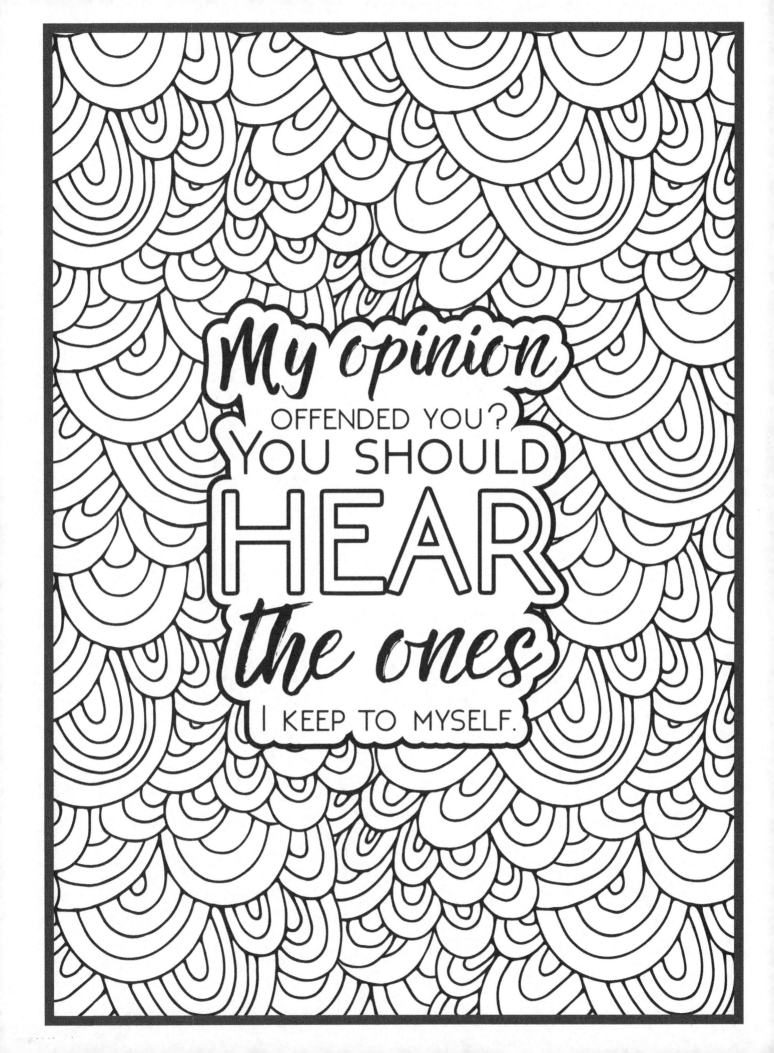

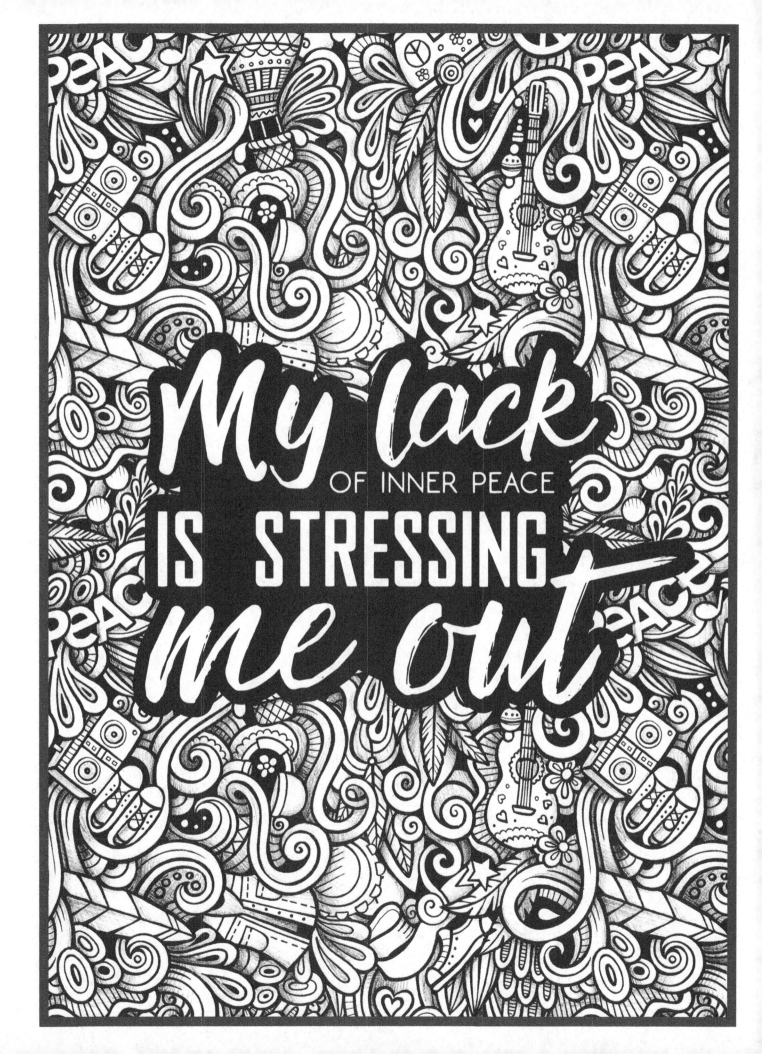

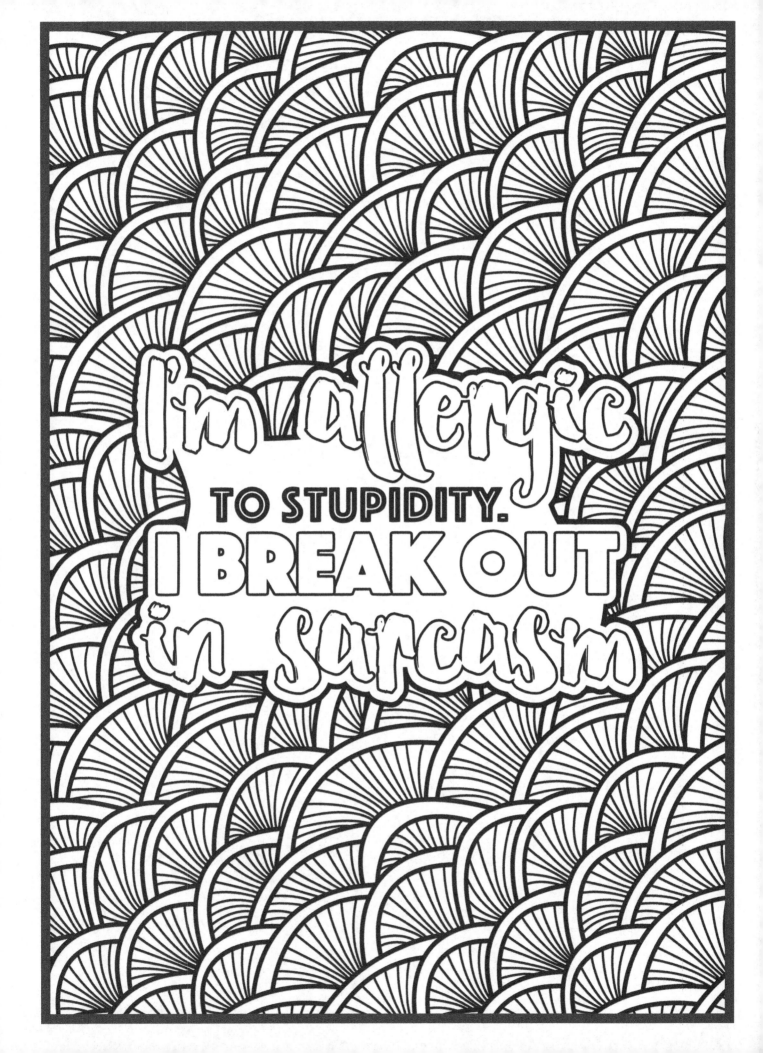

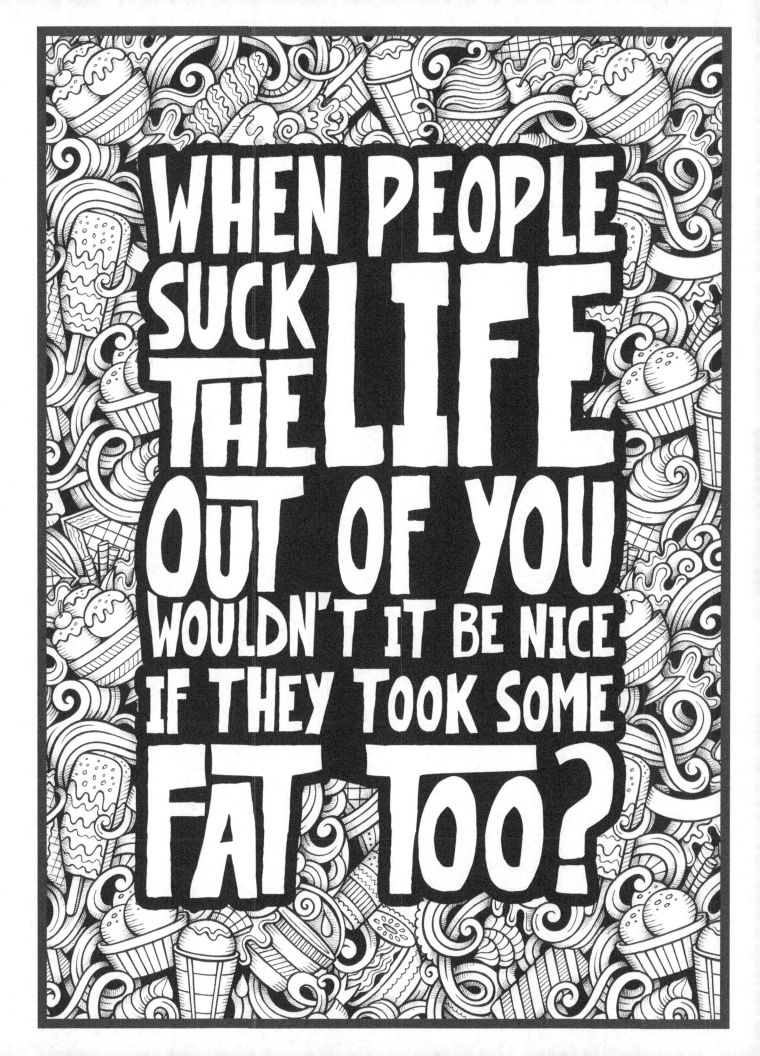

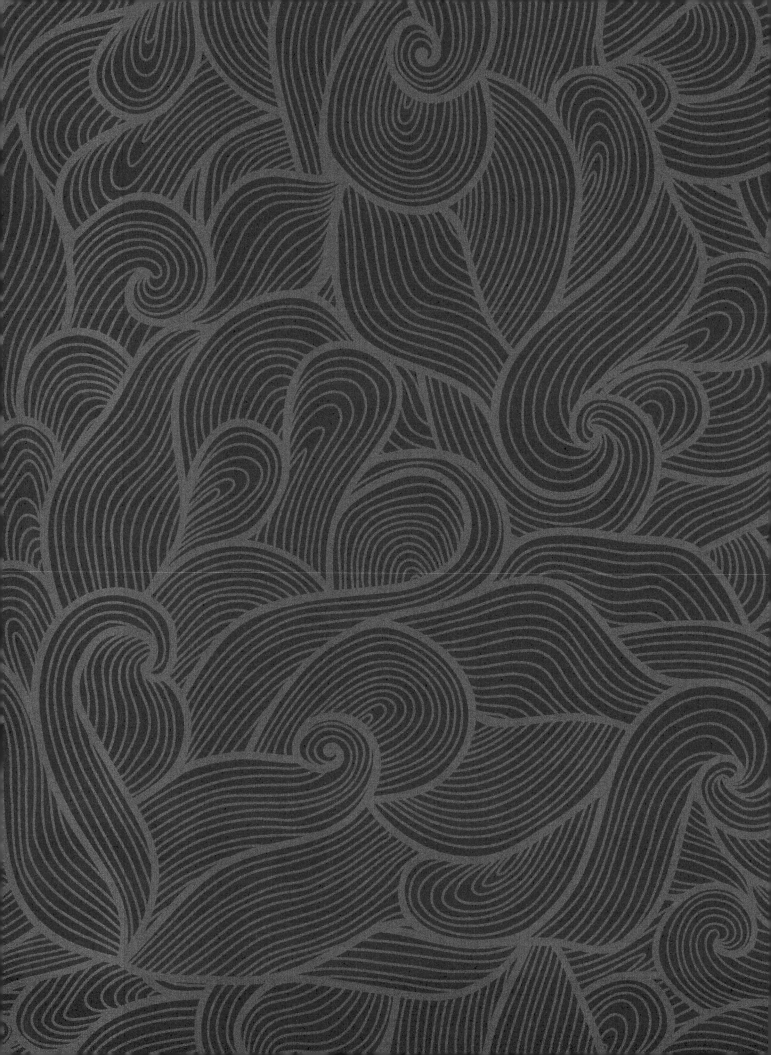

FREEBIE!

JOIN OUR VIP NEWSLETTER AND RECEIVE A FREE DIGITAL DOWNLOAD OF A PRINTABLE PDF <u>ACTIVITY BOOK FOR ADULTS</u> FEATURING INSPIRATIONAL QUOTE COLORING PAGES, MANDALAS, WORD SEARCHES, AND MAZES FOR ADULTS.

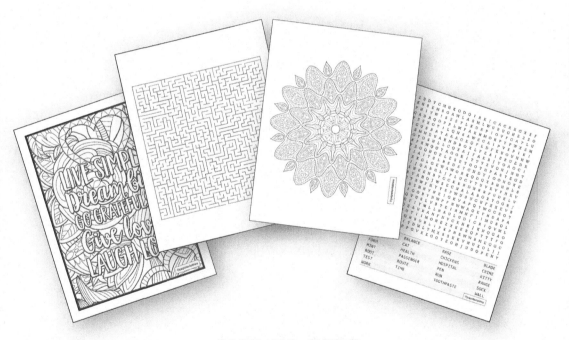

SIGN UP HERE

http://freebies.papeteriebleu.com/FRB3

@papeteriebleu

Papeterie Bleu

Shop our other books at
www.pbleu.com

Wholesale distribution through Ingram Content Group
www.ingramcontent.com/publishers/distribution/wholesale

For questions and customer service, email us at
support@pbleu.com

Made in the USA
Middletown, DE
24 June 2022

67724395R00060